CLINICAL
BLADDER CANCER

CLINICAL BLADDER CANCER

Edited by

L. DENIS

A. Z. Middelheim
Antwerp, Belgium

P. H. SMITH

St. James University Hospital
Leeds, England

and

M. PAVONE-MACALUSO

University Polyclinic Hospital
Palermo, Italy

PLENUM PRESS • NEW YORK AND LONDON

Library of Congress Cataloging in Publication Data

International Symposium on Bladder Cancer (1980 : Antwerp, Belgium)
    Clinical bladder cancer.

    Proceedings of an International Symposium on Bladder Cancer and a
selection of urological papers presented at the Antwerp Medical Days, held
September 19-20, 1980, in Antwerp, Belgium''—Verso t.p.
    The meeting was sponsored by the Antwerp Medical Days Program Com-
mittee.
    Bibliography: p.
    Includes index.
    1. Bladder—Cancer—Congresses. I. Denis, L. II. Smith, P. H. (Philip Henry)
III. Pavone-Macaluso, M. IV. Antwerp Medical Days Program Committee. V.
Title. [DNLM: 1. Bladder neoplasms—Congresses. WJ 504 C641 1980]
RC280.B5I527   1980   616.99′462   81-15855
ISBN-13: 978-1-4613-3355-5   e-ISBN-13: 978-1-4613-3353-1

DOI: 10.1007/978-1-4613-3353-1
                                                                AACR2

Proceedings of an international symposium on bladder cancer and a selection of urological papers presented at the Antwerp Medical Days, held
September 19-20, 1980, in Antwerp, Belgium

© 1982 Plenum Press, New York

Softcover reprint of the hardcover 1st edition 1982

A Division of Plenum Publishing Corporation
233 Spring Street, New York, N.Y. 10013

35th ANTWERP MEDICAL DAYS - SEPTEMBER 18 - 20, 1980

INTERNATIONAL SYMPOSIUM "BLADDER CANCER"

Under the auspices of the Honorable A. Kinsbergen, Governor
of the Province of Antwerp, the Symposium was organized by
THE ANTWERP MEDICAL DAYS.

Program Committee:

L. DENIS	President, Vrije Universiteit Brussel
L. EYCKMANS	President Elect, Institute of Tropical Medicine, Antwerp
P. NOWE	Secretary, A.Z. Middelheim, Antwerpen

Scientific Committee:

P. AUVRAY	President Société Belge d'Urologie
F. EDSMYR	Director World Health Organisation Collaborating Centres for Research and Treatment of Urinary Bladder Cancer
W. GEPTS	Vrije Universiteit Brussel
A. HUBENS	Universitaire Instelling Antwerpen
G. PARIZEL	Universitaire Instelling Antwerpen
M. PAVONE	President EORTC Urological Group
P. SMITH	Secretary EORTC Urological Group
K. VAN CAMP	President Belgische Vereniging voor Urologie.

PREFACE

This volume is a report of the proceedings of an International
Symposium on Bladder Cancer and a selection of Urological papers
presented at the Antwerp Medical Days in Antwerp, Belgium, on the
19th and 20th September 1980. The meeting was sponsored by the
Antwerp Medical Days Program Committee supported by the Royal Antwerp
Circle of Medicine, the Urological Group of the European Organization
for Research on the Treatment of Cancer, the Belgische Vereniging
voor Urologie, the Société Belge d'Urologie, the Province and City of
Antwerp and the National Fund for Scientific Medical Research of
Belgium.

Contributors were briefed to avoid too much overlapping, in the
hope of obtaining a coherent compilation of clinical data. We are
grateful for their discipline which enables early publication.

All the contributions in this volume, except the section on
immunology which was selected by the editors for its related interest, were presented at the International Symposium under the sections
'Understanding the Disease', 'Therapeutic Approaches'. 'Chemotherapy',
and 'Prospective Studies'.

Although the symposium was prepared and the material collected
in Antwerp, it is only proper to acknowledge that the correction of
the manuscripts and the typing of the material was performed in
Leeds. We should particularly like to acknowledge our gratitude to
Mrs. S. Conyers, Miss M. Calder, Mrs. S. Purdie and Miss S. Stevenson
of the Departments of Urology and Oncology of St. James's University
Hospital, Leeds, for their great care and patience in typing this
volume and to the Department of Medical Photography at St. James's
University Hospital for the preparation of Figures 1, 2, 3 and 4
on pages 129-138.

CONTENTS

CONTENTS

INTRODUCTION

L DENIS

Department of Urology
A.Z. Middelheim, Antwerp
Belgium

Bladder cancer constitutes an increasing proportion of malignant disease in the general population. This factor, and its poor prognosis in a substantial number of cases, makes it the biggest challenge to the practising urologist. The major problem is that bladder cancer is a heterogeneous disease whose biological potential shows great variation even within tumors of transitional cell type, which represent almost all clinical bladder cancers in the western hemisphere. Only the histopathologist is able to make the diagnosis and to determine the characteristics which allow a classification of the different varieties of bladder cancer. This diagnosis is based on clinical material provided by the urologist. General agreement exists that this material should include the tumor proper, a "deep bite" after resection of all visible tumor, the adjacent mucosa and selected biopsies from normal looking mucosa. This assessment allows clinical staging and grading, the first and most important step towards proper therapy.

This dependence on a surgical biopsy does not decrease the clinical importance of urinary cytology. Indeed cytology of routine or bladder wash specimens represents our "best bet" for early diagnosis of recurrence after treatment, for the diagnosis of upper tract malignancies, and for the diagnosis of in situ lesions invisible to the eye.

Most patients present with superficial lesions at the time of initial diagnosis. The clinical problems relate to prognosis and more specifically to recurrence, new occurrence, and invasion of the bladder wall. Category Ta lesions are usually not difficult to treat but the Tis (carcinoma in situ) and the T1 lesion may require early aggressive or combination treatment. Patients with invasive

1

and/or distant disease need further evaluation for N and M staging.
Computed tomography lacks precision for accurate T staging but has
proved to be invaluable in providing bidimensional measurements of
abdominal masses. Progress in the development of transurethral
ultrasound may help to solve the perennial problem of understaging
local invasive disease. The definition of the N category remains
an open problem, especially in treatment options where surgical
staging is avoided.

Imperfect as our staging system may be, it is of vital importance in clinical urology for the selection of treatment and comparison of results. The data contributing to clinical and pathological staging form the scientific basis of all treatment in urological oncology. Surgery as the exclusive treatment of bladder
cancer, especially of the invasive lesion, is considered of doubtful
value. Combination treatments combining surgery with radiotherapy
or chemotherapy are evaluated and have shown some promising results.
Unfortunately conflicting data generate uncertainty and, whilst the
advances in chemotherapeutic treatment in both superficial and
invasive bladder cancer have provided some answers, they have
generated even more questions.

One question that remains unanswered is the relationship between
the immune system of the host and the biological potential of the
tumor. A hopeful opening in this direction is the importance of the
presence or absence of normal ABO (H) antigens on the surface of
bladder tumors. The overall assessment of the immune response awaits
further basic studies.

Within this framework, progress in treatment is slow and controversial advice is available on almost every aspect of this complex
problem. The clinician has to choose for his patient between the
Scylla of the natural history of the disease and the Charybdis of
treatment which may be debilitating and at times unnecessary.
Probably the only hope and assurance of the development of adequate
treatment in the presence of such conflicting data is by particip-
ation in controlled clinical trials. The reward for those who so
commit themselves is likely to be slow but steady progress towards
the understanding and the optimal treatment of this dangerous disease.

UNDERSTANDING THE DISEASE

CHAIRMAN'S SUMMARY

J AUVERT

Department of Urology
Hôpital Henri Mondor
Paris, France

Bladder cancers present a major problem to the Urologist, which I must admit, is still far from being solved.

From an etiological point of view, with the increase in cigarette smoking, we see this cancer increasingly commonly in men over 50 and now also in women who are smoking more and more.

Screening has made certain progress with the study of urinary cytology. At the same time we cannot deny that reading the slides is difficult and there are few competent Cytologists. Cytology is making rapid progress for it is even possible to measure intra-cellular DNA levels by cytophotometry and to deduce the degree of malignancy from it. But this is a very elaborate technique requiring a computer and few centres have the appropriate equipment.

The rule for confirming the diagnosis and determining the treatment from the results of transurethral deep biopsies is widely adopted although one still sees some tumours which have only ever been treated by diathermy.

The TNM classification is widely known in Europe. Unfortunately the N category can only be correctly assessed on the data from lymph node resection. The T category is not always perfectly assessed in the clinic or by endoscopy. The CT scan gives a precise measurement of the size of the tumour and its connection with the rectum and the pelvic wall; it is now one of the usual investigations performed before total cystectomy. Similar information can be obtained from ultra-sound by intravesical probe, as demonstrated by Professor Niijima. The G category must be carefully defined as it is of great prognostic value, just as is the architecture, the

degree of invasion of the sub-mucosa and the muscle, the inflammatory reaction, mitoses, metaplasia, intravascular emboli and
the number of sites of tumours. These many elements allow one to
develop a histoprognostic index giving indications on the radio-
sensitivity and the probable rate of survival.

Endovesical chemotherapy in multiple superficial recurrent
tumours is being studied, but its effectiveness would appear slight.
Radium in Holland, radioactive iodine in America and iridium in
France have been used for interstitial radiotherapy. This last
technique is effective in the treatment of solitary medium-sized
tumours (less than 4 cm) of the mobile portion of the bladder.

High Energy Radiation alone is used on 20% of tumours. It is
seen to reduce the N category in many large tumours or, even better,
has an adjuvant effect before cystectomy (30 to 45 grays in 3 to 4
weeks or twice 650 rads -"flash"- over 2 days).

Total cystectomy is useful but can realistically be performed
without too great a risk only in those patients under 70 in
reasonable health and if few lymph nodes are invaded (N1 +). There
is a developing trend to use cutaneous ureterostomy because the
Bricker technique has limited advantages. If the tumour is confined
to the bladder (T2, T3 and N0), one can consider a reconstruction,
after excision, of a reservoir with the sigmoid, the caecum or the
ileum, joined to the apex of the prostate or to the posterior
urethra.

Multiple chemotherapy lasting 6 months is certainly effective
in cases of bone or lung metastases. Agents used alone or together
include Adriamycin, VM 26, Mitomycin-C, 5 FU and in the EORTC
Protocol 30771, Adriamycin, Cyclophosphamide and Cis platinum.

In conclusion, we must say that hematuria in a patient over 50
demands urography, and whether a bladder tumour is shown or not,
endoscopy with a biopsy of the bladder mucosa. Only in this way
can tumours be dectected at a stage when they are still curable.

SOME ASPECTS OF THE PATHOLOGY OF BLADDER CANCER

C K ANDERSON

Department of Pathology
University of Leeds
ENGLAND

INTRODUCTION

Carcinoma of the urinary bladder is a disease of uncertain
natural history with tumours of comparable grade and stage behaving
in quite different ways. A patient with bladder cancer may also
develop homologous tumours at any point in the urinary tract lined
by transitional epithelium.

Mucosal and superficially invasive tumours are best managed by
endoscopic resection and such growths may be successfully treated in
this manner for years only to escape eventually from control. Unfortunately, no single investigation, or group of tests, can unfailingly
predict the effectiveness of any given treatment in any particular
patient, while the commonly used therapeutic modes have not produced
a significant improvement in morbidity and mortality over the last
30 years.

The incidence of bladder cancer is rising in most urban popu-
lations probably due to exposure to industrial carcinogens. There
is a general male to female ratio of about 2.5 : 1, but in some
communities with a high proportion of female workers in long-term
employment, the ratio may fall significantly.

The disease increases in frequency with increasing age and older
patients, up to the end of the eighth decade, have a higher proportion
of poorly differentiated, invasive tumours compared with younger
patients.

PATHOLOGY

     Pathological examination of bladder tumours comprises four
stages.   First, an overall assessment of the nature of the lesion
to determine whether it is truly neoplastic or merely inflammatory,
or reactive.

     Secondly, if it is neoplastic, then the cell type is identified.
The vast majority of bladder tumours are of transitional cell type,
occasionally with metaplastic squamous and glandular areas.   Pure
squamous carcinoma accounts for less than 1% of all tumours seen,
while adenocarcinoma is rarer still.

     Thirdly, an assessment is made of the degree of cellular
differentiation.   This is synonymous with the tumour grade and
describes how closely the tumour cells resemble the putative parent
epithelium.   In the histology report the pathologist describes the
cellular morphology as he sees it, stating whether it is perfectly
differentiated or whether there is loss of differentiation ending in
anaplasia (Table 1).   The TNM "G" grading system is widely used but
the system of Bergkvist et al (2) is sensitive to varying degrees of
de-differentiation and is highly reproducible.

TABLE 1

CELLULAR DIFFERENTIATION IN BLADDER TUMOURS

Histological Appearances	TNM "G" Grade	Grade of Bergkvist et al
Tumour composed of transitional epithelium of normal thickness and cellular appearance.	0	0
Some thickening of the transitional epithelium comprising the tumour, but cells do not deviate significantly from normal.	1	1
The epithelium is thickened and displays moderate cellular irregularity with some variation in nuclear and cellular size.	2	2
There is a marked cellular deviation from normal although the transitional character of the epithelium is preserved. Cells and nuclei vary greatly in size and shape.	3	3
Gross anaplasia with complete loss of transitional epithelial characteristics.	3	4

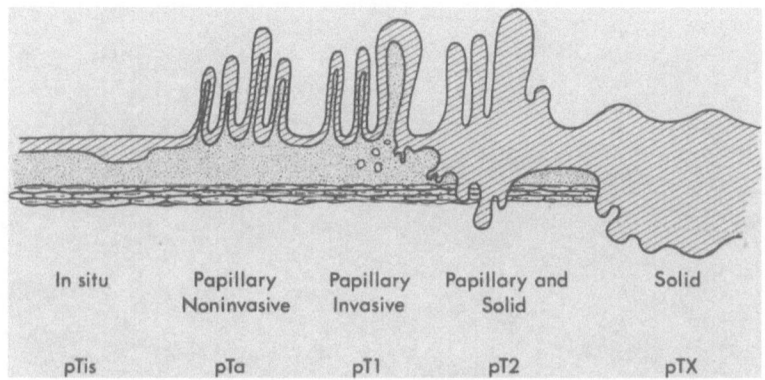

Fig. 1.   Growth Patterns in Bladder Carcinoma.

Finally, the overall growth pattern of the lesion is described
and this is a part, but not the whole, of the staging procedure.
The lesion is categorised as in situ, (fig. 1) pure papillary without
invasion, or solid, which is the British way of describing infiltrating lesions.   The extent of the invasion is established, where this
is possible, and lymphatic permeation is carefully looked for.   The
sub-group tumours described as "papillary and solid" have a very
poor prognosis.   A "papilloma" to be so described must be flawlessly
differentiated and at no point more than seven cell layers thick.

HISTOLOGY

The exophytic outline of inflammatory polypoid cystitis can be
differentiated from a true papillary neoplasm, while solid reactive
lesions, such as cystitis cystica and nephro-genic adenoma, are not
to be confused with the pattern of a true solid tumour.

Transitional cell tumours vary from those showing good differentiation with large surface cells (fig. 2) through varying degrees of
de-differentiation corresponding to Bergkvist Grade 1, 2 and 3 (figs.
3 and 4) to the completely anaplastic.   The true squamous cell
carcinoma with keratinisation and the rare adenocarcinoma can be
readily diagnosed.

The overall growth pattern of papillary tumours is examined to
detect the presence of invasion and its extent.   Superficially
invasive tumours can be readily controlled by skilled endoscopic
resection.   The papillary and solid carcinoma (fig. 5) shows obvious
intracavitary papillary outgrowth with the considerable element of
invasion which makes resection more difficult.

Solid tumours may be merely micro-invasive but usually they
extend deeply into muscle (fig. 6).   Any invasive tumour may produce
lymphatic permeation.

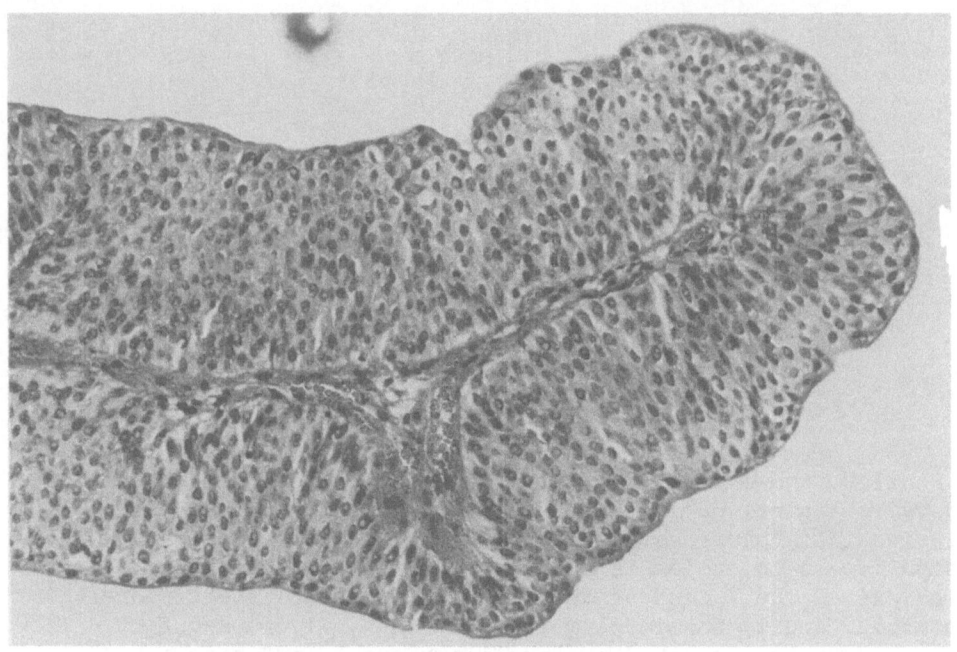

Fig. 2.   Well Differentiated Transitional Cell Carcinoma (Grade 2).
           H and E x 160. Figures 2-7 have been reduced 35% for
           reproduction.

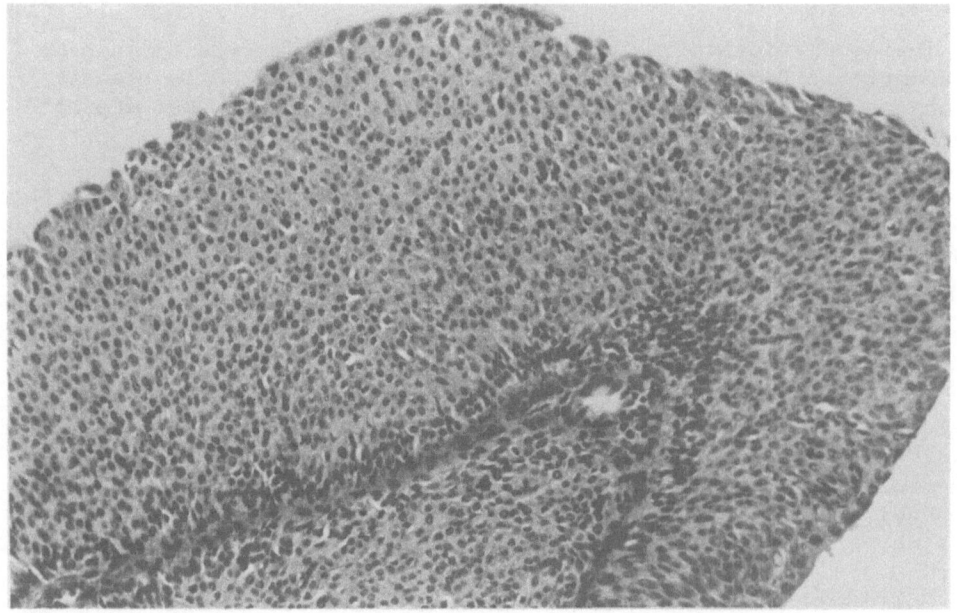

Fig. 3.   Intermediate Transitional Cell Carcinoma (Grade 2).
           H and E x 160

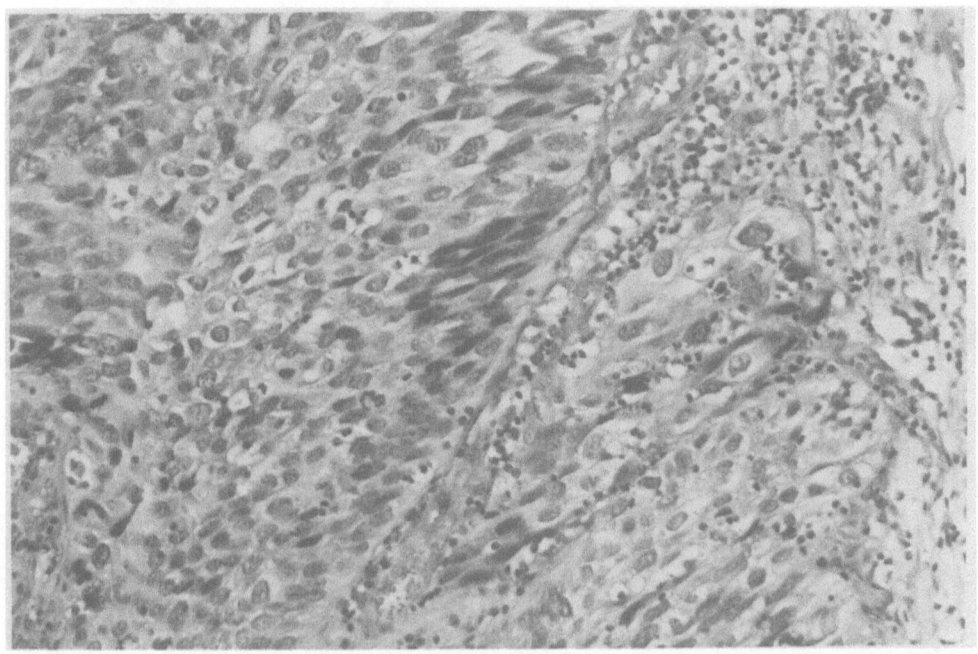

Fig. 4.   Poorly Differentiated Transitional Cell Carcinoma with
          Invasion (Grade 3).   H and E x 160

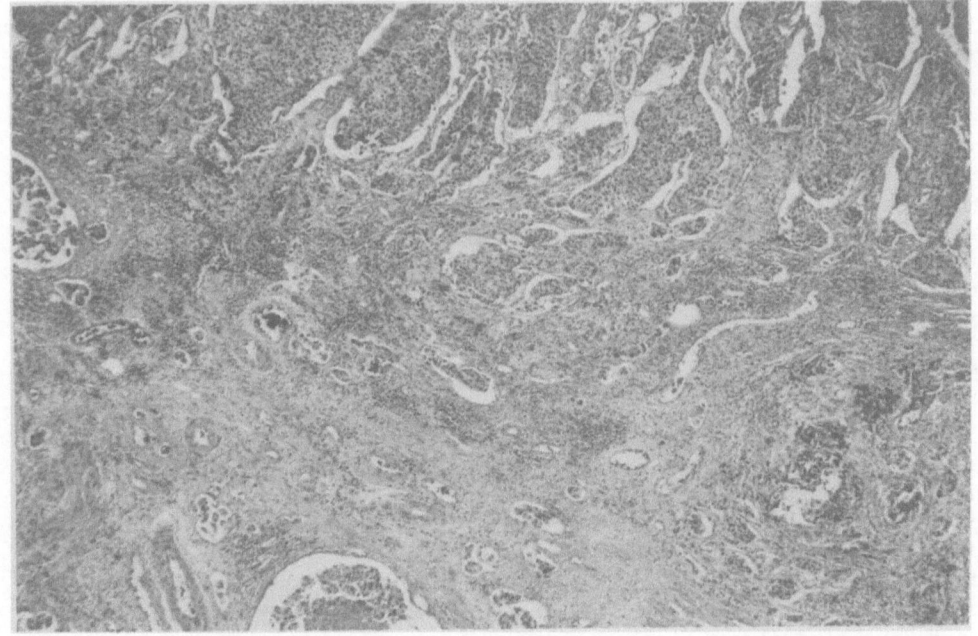

Fig. 5.   Papillary and Solid Carcinoma with a Papillary Element at
          the Top and Invasion into Muscle Beneath.   H and E x 63

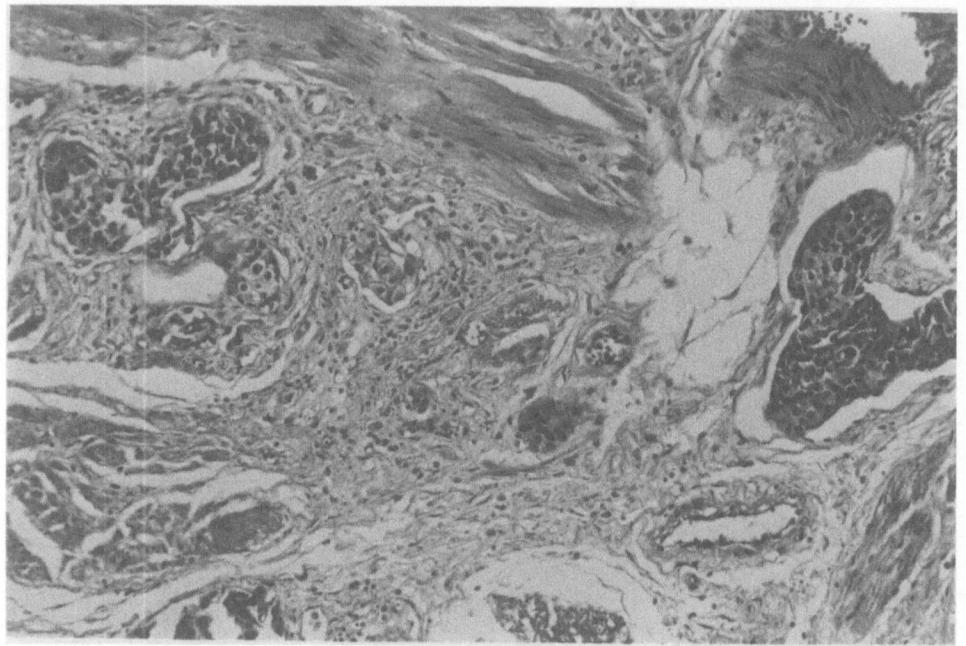

Fig. 6.   Solid, Undifferentiated Carcinoma (Grade 3) Invading
           Muscle.   H and E x 160

CARCINOMA IN SITU

    Carcinoma in situ presents no problem in histological diagnosis
although dysplasia due to inflammatory change may be mistaken for it
(fig. 7).   The majority of patients are males in the sixth and
seventh decades, and of those with symptoms, 65% will develop
invasive or micro-invasive carcinoma within three years.   In the
remainder the lesion persists without obvious progression while in
a small proportion the appearances regress either spontaneously or
after treatment.

MULTIFOCAL TUMOURS

    The multifocal nature of bladder carcinoma is frequently
stressed.   There may be several synchronous tumours at the first
clinical presentation, while after successful primary treatment,
successive generations of tumour arise.   These are generally of
comparable histology and invasive potential to the primary.   Large
invasive tumours are often accompanied and adjoined by areas of
carcinoma in situ and by smaller tumours well separated from the main
primary.   In addition, tumours may also develop in the renal pelvis,
ureter and the urethra.   Despite this one sees solitary invasive
carcinoma in cystectomy specimens where the remainder of the bladder

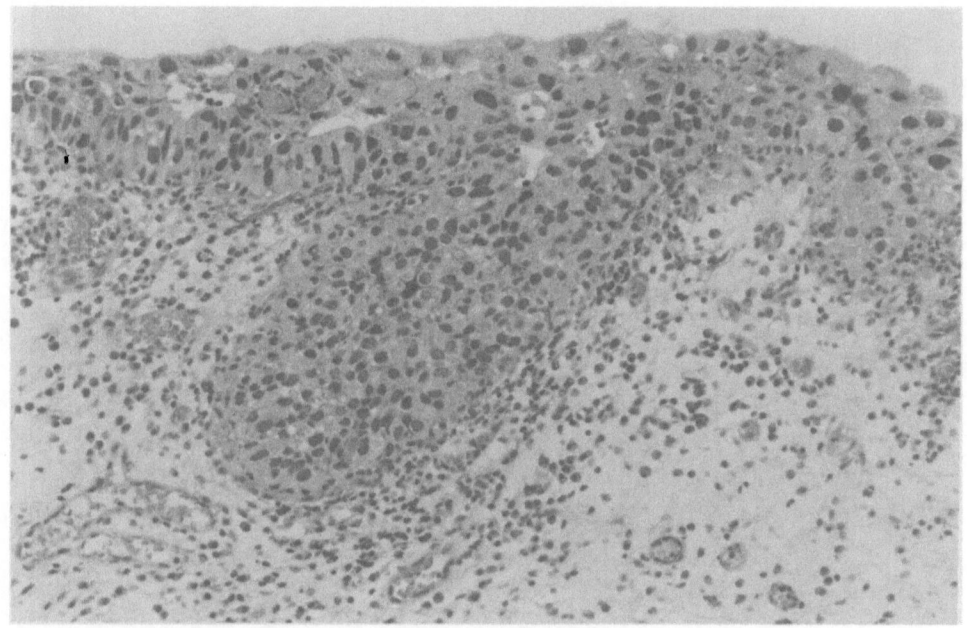

Fig. 7.   Carcinoma in Situ.   H and E x 160

mucosa appears histologically normal and patients treated by
cystectomy alone may remain free of tumour in the upper tract and
residual urethra for many years.   It is possible that there are two
forms of tumour generation, one arising in a localised area of epithelial transformation and another arising after extensive field
pre-malignant change has taken place in the urinary tract.   Transitional cell carcinoma in the prostatic ducts (fig. 8) is a real
challenge to the urologist and can often be successfully managed by
resection.   On the other hand, invasion of the prostate by bladder
carcinoma (pT4) is usually rapidly fatal.

SPREAD OF BLADDER CARCINOMA

     Bladder cancer spreads by direct invasion and lymphatic borne
metastases.   More rarely haematogeneous spread occurs following
vascular invasion (fig. 9).

     Direct invasion occurs into the stromal cores of the fronds of
papillary tumours and into the lamina propria in both papillary and
solid growths.   Superficial lymphatic permeation takes place at this
point facilitating deeper and wider spread and accounting for the
uncommon, but well documented phenomenon of a superficial tumour
producing distant metastases.

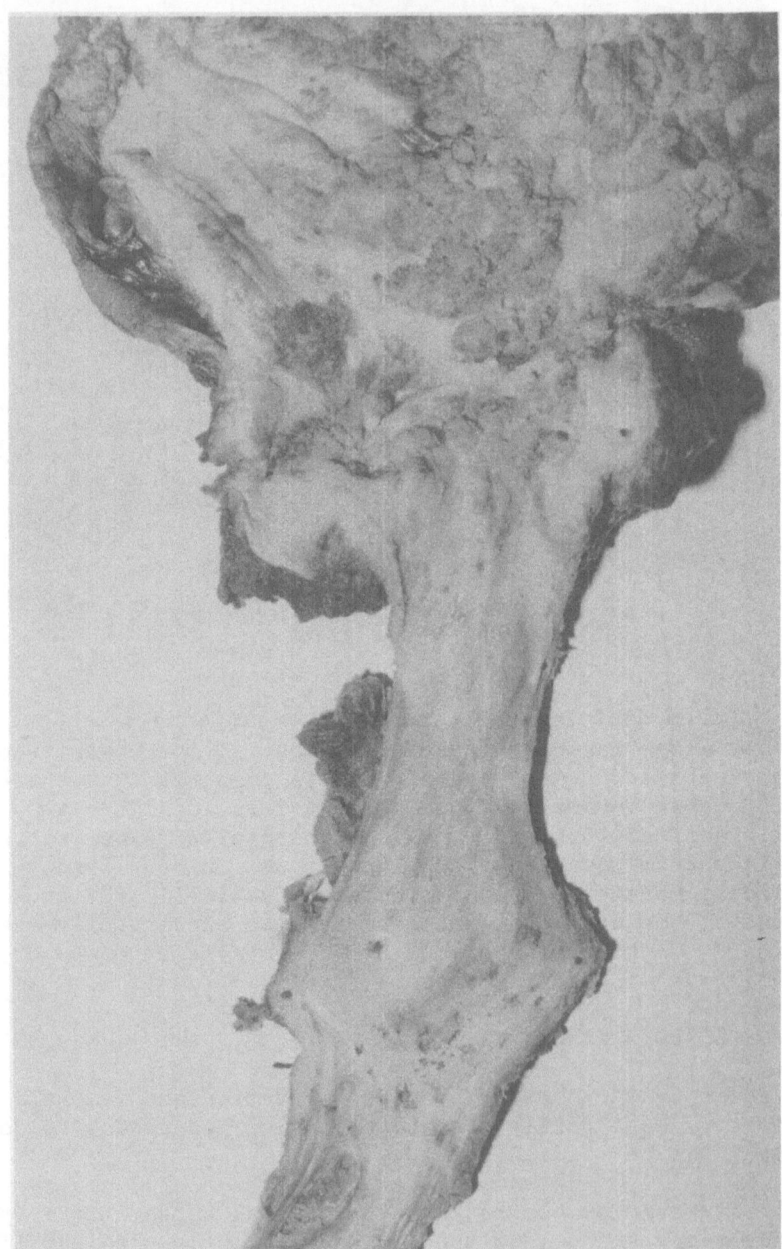

Fig. 8.   Papillary Invasive Carcinoma in the Bladder with Tumours
           in the Prostatic and Penile Urethra.

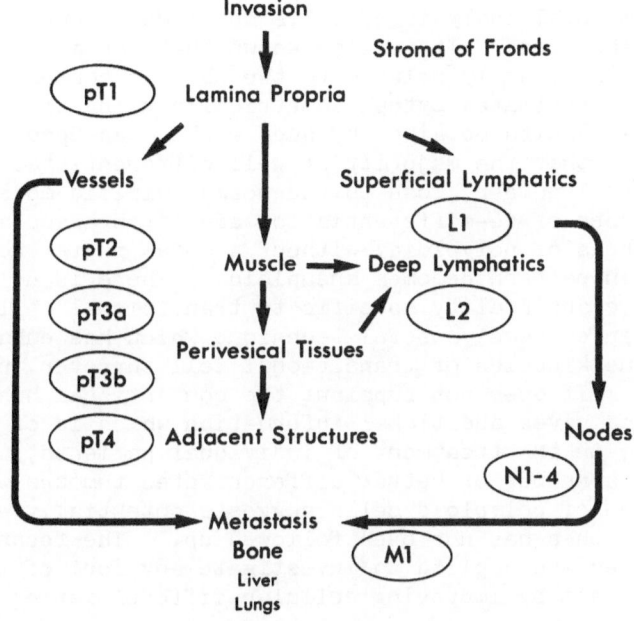

Fig. 9.   Spread of Bladder Carcinoma.

Deeper invasion infiltrates and destroys the muscle extending through the wall of the bladder to the perivesical tissues.   Anderson (1) showed that, in a series of patients with treated bladder carcinoma coming to post-mortem examination, pelvic malignant disease was the principal cause of death in 60%.   This was due to a combination of local extension and particularly lymphatic involvement below the pelvic brim.

Hepatic and pulmonary metastases were of less importance but 78% of advanced cases had bone metastases and in 38% of patients bone pain was the first symptom indicating treatment failure and tumour dissemination.

ADDITIONAL METHODS OF PATHOLOGICAL EXAMINATION

Chromosomal Changes

It is to be expected that rapidly proliferating tumours and areas of unstable mucosa will develop nuclear karyotypic abnormalities commensurate with the degree of cellular de-differentiation.   The cells used for this estimation can be taken by endoscopic biopsy or from freshly voided urine and the hypothesis has been proved valid

by direct chromosomal analysis of cells in mitosis, but the technique
is extremely laborious.   It is also known that the amount of chromosomal material is directly related to the nuclear content of DNA and
that this can be estimated cytophotometrically using the Feulgen
reaction.   The results obtained by such workers as Spooner and
Cooper (5) prove that the majority of well differentiated tumours
have a chromosomal number close to the normal diploid mode of 46.
Increasing degrees of de-differentiation are often associated with
increasing degrees of polyploidy without a modal preference until
the distribution pattern becomes aneuploid.   There is no characteristic karyotypic abnormality specific to transitional cell carcinoma.
This has been an extremely useful technique which has enhanced our
knowledge of the kinetics of transitional cell turnover, proliferation
and neoplasia.   It does not supplant the conventional histological
grade and seldom gives additional information which is of immediate
practical value in the treatment of individual patients, although
the finding of a number of better differentiated tumours with an
increased number of polyploid cells suggests potentially enhanced
malignancy, but this has not been followed up.   The technique could
always be revived and applied to investigate any form of therapy
which claims to act by improving cellular differentiation.

Electron Microscopy

The appearance of tumour cells as seen by transmission electron
microscope have been classically described by Fulker (3).   There is
disruption of the surface membrane which is thrown into microvilli.
Tight junctions are poorly formed and the intercellular relationships
are disturbed by the formation of spaces often containing microvilli.
The appearnces of marker chromosomes is a clear indication of neoplastic transformation.   There is a marked increase in papillary
vessels in the lamina propria.   The scanning electron microscope
shows surface changes in the tumour cells with greater facility re-
vealing varying degrees of villus formation, cellular cobblestoning
and imperfect cellular apposition.   It is often difficult to know
whether these cellular appearances are a reflection of basic alteration in structure specific to the process of neoplastic transformation, or whether they merely represent changes consequent upon rapid
cellular proliferation.   Electron microscopy, therefore, does not
reveal the potential of a given bladder tumour or an area of epithelium with a certainty which makes its use mandatory in all cases.

Tissue Culture

Transitional cell tumours can be successfully cultured using
a suitable medium or nutrient matrix.   Under these circumstances
tumours of the same grade produce widely different growth patterns
(4).   The reason for this fascinating variation is presently unknown
and its significance is not fully understood but the technique could
prove of considerable value both as an expression of cellular growth

potential and as a means of testing the effects of environmental change on a particular tumour.

CONCLUSION

Because of the extreme clinical importance of bladder cancer and of the intellectual challenge offered by access to sequential biopsies from the same patient the histopathologist will continue to apply to such material every new technique available.   In so doing he must beware of circumlocution - of expressing the same judgement in more elaborate and less readily comprehensible form.

The carefully selected and skilfully taken biopsy remains the stock in trade of the histopathologist and all such material should be examined with scrupulous attention to detail.   In performing this pedestrian task the histopathologist may impart information which is of real value in patient management and his simple assessment will act as an invaluable control of more complex and expensive forms of examination.

REFERENCES

1.   C.K. Anderson, Current Topics on the Pathology of Bladder
      Cancer, Proc. Royal Soc. Med., 66: 283 (1973).
2.   A. Bergkvist, A. Ljungqvist and G. Moberger, Classification of
      Bladder Tumours Based on Cellular Pattern, Acta Chirurgica
      Scandinavica, 130: 371 (1965).
3.   M.J. Fulker, E.H. Cooper and T. Tanaka, Proliferation and
      Ultrastructure of Papillary Transitonal Cell Carcinoma of the
      Human Bladder, Cancer 27: 71 (1971).
4.   J. Leighton, N. Abaza, R. Tchao, K. Geisinger and J. Valentich,
      Development of Tissue Culture Procedures for Predicting the
      Individual Risk of Recurrence of Bladder Cancer, Cancer Res.
      37: 2854 (1977).
5.   M.E. Spooner and E.H. Cooper, Chromosome Constitution of
      Transitional Cell Carcinoma of the Urinary Bladder.   Cancer
      29: 1401 (1972).

URINARY CYTOLOGY TODAY

H J de VOOGT, J S PLOEM, J A M BRUSEE and C F H M KNEPFE

Department of Cyto- and Histochemistry
State University at Leiden
Holland

Urinary cytology has significantly contributed to the diagnosis of bladder cancer. More specifically, it has enhanced the diagnostic yield of carcinoma-in-situ (8). It has improved prognostic grading and it has an important place in the follow-up of treated bladder cancer patients. The reliability of urinary cytology has been confirmed in numerous scientific contributions (7). In this connection it is worth noting here once again the specify and sensitivity of cytology of smears of sediment of fresh voided urine samples, stained by Papanicolaou and/or Giemsa stains (2).

In those cases where the yield of cells is small or when the methods of sampling and fixation or transport can influence the results negatively, the processing of bladder washings may give better results. We use it only very rarely and it should be stressed that it can be done with physiological saline only, because other fluids more often than not cause artefacts. Preparatory techniques are described in detail esewhere (2).

The question remains: is it possible to improve the results any further?

In recent years quantitative cytology has been introduced, whereby objective parameters such as nuclear morphometry, DNA and RNA content and chromatin texture are analysed and used for refinement and standardisation of cytologic diagnosis as well as for automation of cytology. For instance a taxonomic intra-cellular analytic system was developed by Wied et al (9) in which a computer could identify digitized cell images. Koss et al (5) applied this system to urothelial cells with success.

Much simpler are the methods by which DNA or RNA are stained quantitatively by fluorescent stains such as Feulgen and acridine-orange. After the staining procedure cells can be rapidly passed through apparatus, in which DNA-values of cells are measured by flow and pulse-cytophotometry (6). By measuring fluorescence of the nuclei in this way, tumorcells with more than diploid DNA-values can be recognised, or histograms of a given cell-suspension can be made. These systems work with only one objective parameter. This is also the case in nuclear morphometry in which the surface area of nuclei are measured by means of a so-called X-Y-tablet and a small computer, and the nuclei of normal and abnormal cells can be compared statistically.

In Leyden the department of histo- and cytochemistry has worked on the automation of cytology, initially aimed to assist with cervical cytology. However it proved to be suitable for urinary cytology as well.

First a two-color fluorescence staining procedure was developed (4). DNA is quantitatively stained by Acriflavine - Feulgen and proteins in cytoplasm are stained semi-quantitatively by Stilbene-Iso-Thyo-cyanotodi-Sulfonic acid (SITC), together called the AFS-stain. By using an MPV-microscope with dichroic mirrors for two-wavelength excitation, the nuclei can be measured by their yellow fluorescence (Feulgen) and the morphological diagnosis can be made by the blue fluorescence of the cytoplasm. This was done by measuring aselectively 100 cells of a given urinary sediment, as well as by measuring 100 atypical cells after preselection by the analyst. The results can be seen in Fig. 1. They show the histograms of non selected and selected measurements of a grade 1, 2 and 4 tumor of the bladder. Lymphocytes were added for standard 2 C DNA-values (3). In a second study, urines from 203 patients with benign and malignant urothelial diseases were screened and the results show that in all grade 2-4 lesions a relative DNA-value of more than 5C was found. (Table 1). This means that DNA-value can be used as a screening parameter.

The next step was the LEYTAS-computer (Leyden Television Assisted Texture Analysis System), in which nuclear morphometry and cytofluorometry are combined for a fully automated screening of cytologic smears. The absorption image of the AFS-stained smears is scanned by a special microscope with a TV-camera that projects the image on a TV-screen (black and white). The different grey-levels of the plumbicon tube are used for selection of cells by DNA-content of the nuclei and an image transformation procedure (erosion) is used to measure the nucleus. Another transformation procedure (skeletonisation) has the task of finding and rejecting artefacts such as overlapping clusters of cells and dirt particles. Finally all screened cells are counted, and on the basis of the atypical cells found (more than 5 C DNA-fluorescent intensity X nuclear size)

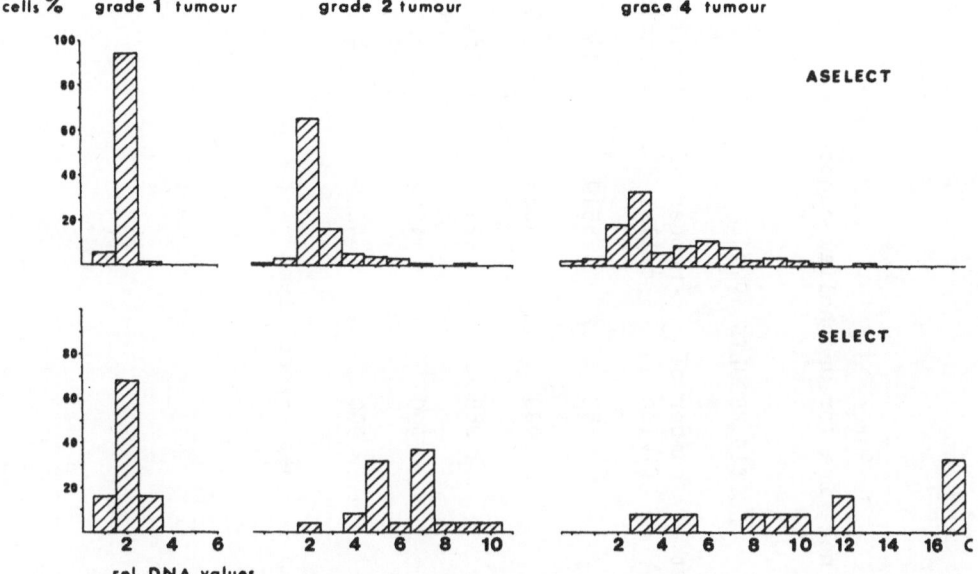

Fig. 1.   The histograms of a grade 1, grade 2 and grade 4 urothelial
          carcinoma after aselect and select DNA cytophotometry. (3)

Table 1
DNA-Values in Urinary Sediment Smears 1975 - 1977

RELATIVE DNA-VALUES

CLINICAL AND/OR HISTOLOGICAL DIAGNOSIS	≤ 5C		5C > < 7C		≥ 7C		TOTAL
	CYT. NEG.	CYT. POS.	CYT. NEG.	CYT. POS.	CYT. NEG.	CYT. POS.	
NORMAL	65	–	2	–	–	–	67
UROLOGICAL COMPLAINTS	56	1	7	1	4	1	70
GRADE 0-1 UROTHELIAL TUMORS	15	–	1	–	1	–	17
GRADE 2, 3 AND 4 UROTHELIAL CA. AD CIS	–	–	2	7	3	37	49
TOTAL	136	1	12	8	8	38	203

Table 2

LEYTAS - screening of urine of 5 patients, negative for urothelial cancer

CYTOLOGY	HISTOLOGY	LEYTAS RESULTS 1979				
		false alarms	suspect cells	number of fields	number of cells	cell-density
NEGATIVE						
negative	-	-	-	652	8519	13
inflammation	f.u. ca. after TUR	2	-	900	4088	4.5
inflammation	-	-	-	1085	12167	18
inflammation	f.u. pap. after TUR	1	-	900	11642	13
inflammation	f.u. pap.	-	-	900	4239	4.7

ca. = bladder cancer   f.u. = follow-up   pap. = papilloma

Table 3

LEYTAS – screening of urine of 15 patients with urothelial carcinoma

LEYTAS RESULTS 1979

CYTOLOGY POSITIVE	HISTOLOGY	false alarms	suspect cells	number of fields	number of cells	cell-density
atypia 3A	atypia	1	1	900	31241	35
atypia 3A	atypia	1	1	500	6047	12
atypia 3A	f.u. ca. after TUR	–	2	900	16580	18
atypia 3B	f.u. ca. after TUR	–	1	1300	13011	10
atypia 3B	f.u. ca. after TUR	1	1	900	32317	36
Pap 4 and 5	ca. confirmed	6	16	150	3599	24
Pap 4 and 5	ca. confirmed	–	4	232	5674	24
Pap 4 and 5	ca. confirmed	4	25	531	32547	61
Pap 4 and 5	ca. confirmed	1	8	313	22282	71
Pap 4 and 5	ca. confirmed	2	11	204	6720	33
Pap 4 and 5	ca. confirmed	6	22	800	80420	100
Pap 4 and 5	ca. confirmed	2	7	400	14851	37
Pap 4 and 5	ca. confirmed	14	13	1068	72617	68
Pap 4 and 5	ca. confirmed	11	21	400	58635	146
Pap 4 and 5	ca. confirmed	1	16	900	22972	25

ca. = bladder cancer   f.u. = follow-up   pap. = papilloma

LEYTAS PROCESSING

PER SLIDE   PER 100 SUSPECT SLIDES

1. AUTOMATIC FOCUSSING   1. REPLAY SUSPECT CELLS FOUND ON
2. PRESELECTION OF SUSPECT CELLS   SLIDE N ON TV-MONITOR ($\pm$ 30
   ON THE BASIS OF DNA OR   CELLS PER DISPLAY)
   CHROMATIN CONTRAST   2. VISUAL INSPECTION FOR
3. AUTOMATIC ARTEFACT REJECTION   CONFIRMATION OF DIAGNOSIS
4. STORAGE OF SUSPECT CELLS   3. ASK FOR MICROSCOPIC FIELD
   LEFT, IN BUFFER MEMORY (16   REPLAY IF NECESSARY (EXECUTED
   GREY VALUES)   AFTER 100 SLIDES HAVE BEEN
5. NEXT FIELD OR EXIT   REVIEWED)

Fig. 2. The technique of LEYTAS processing.

and the number of cells screened, an aytypia index can be computed.
(1).

False alarms can be reevaluated visually since the computer
can replay these from its memory. The LEYTAS processing is shown
in Fig. 2. The results of five negative and fifteen positive
urines are given in tables 2 and 3. Not only is the selection of
malignant cases surprisingly reliable, but also it is clear that cell
density in the suspect and malignant cases is significantly greater
than in the negative cases.

Though the need for automated cytological screening of urinary
sediment is questionable, there is no doubt that this procedure
(quantification of certain elements of visual evaluation) contributes
considerably to standardisation and refinement of urinary cytology.

REFERENCES

1. P.H. Bartels, L.G. Koss, J. Sychra, and G.L. Wied, Indices of
   Cell Atypia in Urinary Tract Cytology, Acta. Cytol. 22: 387
   (1978)
2. M.E. Beyer-Boon, "The efficacy of Urinary Cytology", Thesis,
   Leiden, 1977.
3. M.E. Beyer-Boon, C. Hilgevoord-de Ruyter, J.S. Ploem, and H.J.
   de Voogt, The applicability of Acriflavine-SITS-stain in Urinary
   Cytology, in: "The Automation of Cancer Cytology and Cell Image
   Analysis (Proceedings)," N.J. Pressman and G.L. Wied, ed.,
   Japan, pp 207-211 (1977).
4. C.J. Cornelisse and J.S. Ploem, A New Type of Two-colour
   Fluorescence Staining for Cytology Specimens, J. Histochem.
   Cytochem. 24: 72-81 (1976).

5. L.G. Koss, P.H. Bartels, and L.G. Wied, Computer-based Diagnostic
    Analysis of Cells in the Urinary Sediment, J. Urol. 123: 846
    (1980).
6. B. Tribukait and P.L. Esposti, Quantitative Flow Microfluoro-
    metric Analysis of the DNA in Cells from Neoplasms of the Urinary
    Bladder, Urol. Res. 6: 201 (1978).
7. H.J. De Voogt, M.E. Beyer-Boon and P. Rathert, "Atlas of Urinary
    Cytology," Springer Verlag, Heidelberg, (1977).
8. H.J. de Voogt, Primary and Secondary Carcinoma in situ of the
    Bladder, in: "Prevention and Detections of Cancer," H.E. Nieburgs,
    ed., M. Dekker, New York, part 2, vol. 2, pp 2255-2269 (1980).
9. G.L. Wied, P.H. Bartels, G.F. Bahr, and D.G. Oldfield, Taxonomic
    Intra-cellular Analytic System (TICAS) for Cell Identification,
    Acta. Cytol. 12: 180 (1968).

BLADDER TUMOR - DIAGNOSIS

A STEG

Department of Urology
Hôpital Cochin
Paris, France

INTRODUCTION

Precocity in diagnosing a bladder tumor is certainly one of the most important prognostic factors and one may regret that it is not rare for the tumor to be misdiagnosed and precious time lost.

The typical symptomatology of a bladder tumor is well known. The patient, usually a man, complains of hematuria. At IVP an abnormality is seen on the bladder film and cystoscopy easily demonstrates the tumor whilst transurethral resection (TUR) removes it and allows histologic study.

As the clinical picture is so typical, why is there so often some delay in diagnosis? It may be the fault of the patient who is often neglectful and as bleeding generally stops he does not seek medical care immediately. It may also - and this is more surprising - originate in medical misdiagnosis, whether it is attributed to the physician, to the radiologist, or to the urologist.

Among 199 patients with bladder tumor the delay between first symptoms and first consultation was more than 6 months in one case out of two. Only one third of patients were seen within 3 months.

PITFALLS IN DIAGNOSIS

Let us consider these 3 stages of the diagnosis.

A. When the patient attends his physician there are 3 common errors:
   i. The finding at physical examination of an enlarged prostate;

27

one must be very careful before accepting benign prostatic hyper-
trophy (BPH) as the cause of hematuria.
 ii. Anticoagulant therapy; one must emphasize that even when hypocoagulability is proven hematuria deserves full urological
investigation.
iii. The fact that in 15% of the cases there is no hematuria and
the symptomatology is much less alarming, e.g., cystitis, frequency,
or nocturia. We would like to stress the point that a non responsive
recurrent cystitis is very suspicious, as unexplained frequency and
urgency are the most common symptoms of carcinoma in situ (C.I.S).

B. At the radiological stage there are also many risks of error:
 i. When the lesion is a "carcinoma in situ" the bladder may
appear absolutely normal at cystography.
 ii. The risk of error is more common when the tumor is situated
at the bladder neck, is small (it is particularly important to
examine the bladder when it is half empty) or when the tumor develops
in a diverticulum and when there is a ureterocele.
iii. But the major factor, which in our experience leads most
frequently to error, is the discovery on X-ray of some urologic
abnormality which may be considered - wrongly - as the cause of the
bleeding, such as prostatic lithiasis, BPH, stone, and above all,
renal cyst.

     When a "space occupying lesion" is seen on IVP it quickly
focuses the diagnostic discussion and not enough attention is paid
to the other segments of the urinary tract. We have observed some
disastrous cases. In one, a 68 year old man was operated on for a
left renal cyst because of hematuria. After operation the hematuria
persisted and then a bladder tumor was discovered at cystoscopy. In
a second, a 69 year old man with hematuria was operated on for a
cyst. He died of pulmonary embolism and at post mortem a papilloma
was discovered in the bladder which was the cause of the hematuria.
As renal cysts are extremely frequent we want to underline that an
uncomplicated cyst can never be accepted as the explanation of an
episode of hematuria, and that endoscopic control is mandatory in
the diagnosis of hematuria, even when some kidney abnormality is
discovered at IVP.

C. At the urological stage there is generally no problem and at
cystoscopy the tumor is almost always seen. "Almost always", but
not always. As a matter of fact there are 3 pitfalls:- when there
is marked cystitis, when tumor develops in a diverticulum and when
the tumor is C.I.S. In this last case, some redness, or yellow
dots may be seen but often the bladder lining appears normal. We
experimented and found that the less obvious abnormalities are
more easily discovered when cystoscopy is performed with little
distension and with low intensity of illumination.

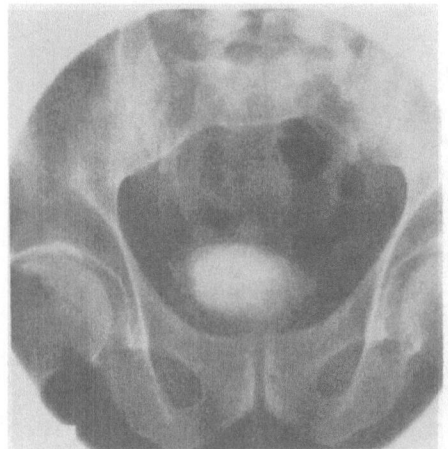

Fig. 1   Irregularity of the left
side of the bladder

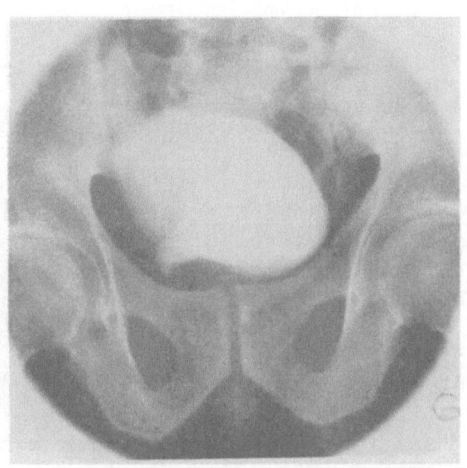

Fig. 2   Same patient as in Fig. 1 –
IVP 18 months later

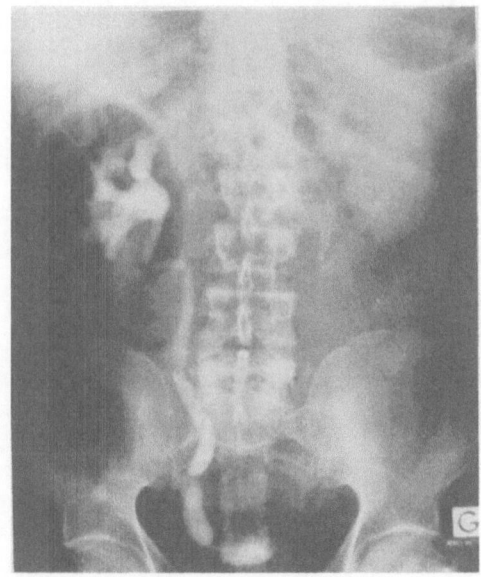

Fig. 3   Stasis in right ureter
attributed to stone

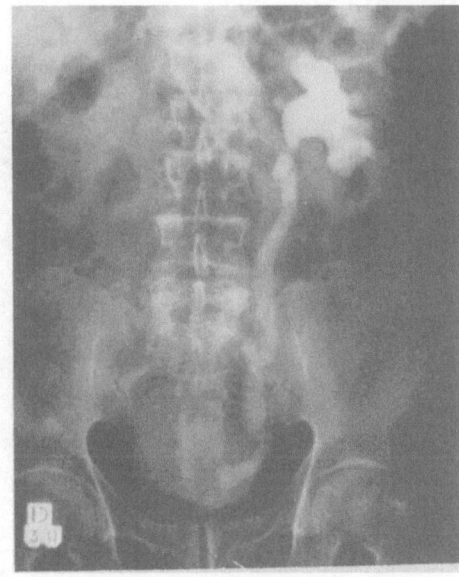

Fig. 4   Same patient as in Fig. 3 –
IVP 18 months later

D. CLINICAL EXAMPLES

One may think that in a meeting with urologists we place too much emphasis on clinical problems, but 3 examples will demonstrate the disastrous consequences of misdiagnosing these tumors.

Mr C., a 56 year old man, complained of hematuria. As he had for many years been treated by anticoagulation therapy, the hematuria was attributed to hypocoagulability. Insufficient attention was paid to the bladder irregularity on IVP (Fig. 1). Eighteen months later the tumor had enlarged considerably (Fig. 2). The man was treated by radical cystectomy and he died 4 months later with general metastases. Mr L., a 54 year old man, complained of right renal colic, hematuria and he passed a uric acid stone. At IVP stasis in the right ureter was attributed to the stone despite the fact that the investigation was performed after the stone had been passed (Fig. 3). Hematuria recurred at intervals and at a second IVP, eighteen months later (Fig. 4), the right kidney was not functioning and the left showed obstruction. Mr L. recently underwent radical cystectomy. When we asked him which type of hematuria he complained of, he described typical terminal hematuria, which obviously could not be explained by a ureteric stone. Mr D., a 67 year old man, complained of frequency by day and night in 1974. One year later these symptoms were attributed to prostatic enlargment and TUR was performed. One year later (1976) supra-pubic-transvesical prostatectomy was carried out. As the symptoms persisted the patient underwent a further TUR in 1977, and twice in 1978. It was only in 1979, six years after the beginning of the trouble that the first cytological examination was performed and malignant cells discovered. TUR biopsy of the bladder demonstrated typical carcinoma in situ (Table 1).

TABLE 1

C.I.S.

D ... M ., ♂, 67

Since 1973	Day and night frequency
1974	T.U.R.P.
1976	Suprapubic transvesical prostatectomy
1977	T.U.R.P.
1978 (March)	Cryosurgery
1978 (April)	Cryosurgery
1979	First cytologic examination

HOW CAN THESE TERRIBLE MISTAKES BE AVOIDED?

The most important rule is that every unexplained urological symptom, and especially hematuria, has to be investigated by clinical, radiological and cystoscopic examination. Two other pieces of advice seem to us to be very important:

i. Use cytological examination generously. As demonstrated by Dr de Voogt, it is the most simple method in diagnosing bladder tumor. It is almost as accurate as cystoscopy; among 255 patients with bladder tumor, we found 90% positive results. It is more accurate than cystoscopy in conditions where carcinoma exists but cannot be seen, e.g., cancer in a diverticulum, cystitis masquerading as bladder tumor and above all C.I.S. One of the main characteristics of C.I.S. is that it exfoliates malignant cells at a high rate.

The only problem is to remember to ask for cytology when the patient complains of frequency, urgency, pain or unexplained "cystitis-like" symptoms. The delay before first cyto-diagnosis is often unbelievably long (2).

ii. The second advice is to use TUR generously when the slightest abnormality is discovered. It is often necessary to repeat this examination. In C.I.S. diagnosis was often made only after 2, 3 or 4 TUR's (Table 2) for all transitions between hyperplasia, dysplasia and C.I.S may be seen and the diagnosis is not always easy. However with these two examinations, cyto-diagnosis and TUR, the diagnosis can hardly be missed.

TUMOR EVALUATION

The demonstration of the presence of a tumor in the bladder is only a small part of the diagnostic problem. What does "bladder tumor" mean? Is it fair to use the same term for a simple pedunculated papilloma as for a vast trigonal infiltrating carcinoma? When should we treat them locally and when by radical surgery?

TABLE 2

16 C.I.S.

Number of T.U.R. performed for diagnosis

1	7 cases
2	4 cases
3	4 cases
4	1 case

The most important factor which indicates the prognosis and
the choice of treatment is staging:
i.   Of the tumor by pathological findings, urography, arteriography,
lymphography, echography, scanning, etc.,
ii. Also of the mucosa at a distance from the tumor since Althausen,
Daly and Prout (3) demonstrated the prognostic significance of such
abnormalities.

Although very important, such "static" staging is not sufficient.
The real problem for the clinician is not the anaplastic tumor of
advanced stage since its potential is well known. The real problem
arises with the well differentiated non invasive tumors or when
invasion does not go beyond the lamina propria. Here, in these very
common tumors, the evolution is not predictable. It is not yet
possible to determine which tumor will never recur and which will
become invasive and fatal. In these circumstances it is also not
possible to decide which tumor should be treated conservatively,
(taking the risk of regretting the decision if the tumor subsequently
becomes invasive), and which radically (taking the risk of an
unnecessary mutilation). Herein lies the basic clinical problem of
the disease.

In this dilemma we now have 2 valuable new guidelines at our
disposal, we can study the "risk factors", and go some way towards
establishing the biological potentiality of the tumor.

The Risk Factors

We did a retrospective study of 199 stage A tumors, where, with
a follow-up of at least 5 years, we knew precisely the "outcome" of
all these cases. And we concluded that some factors may predict
evolution:
i.   The depth of invasion of chorion. The prognosis is different
in Stage A tumor where the chorion is only superficially invaded
(Fig. 5) from that in the A_2 lesion where the chorion is totally
invaded (Fig. 6). Stage A_2 tumors are twice as likely to become
invasive as Stage A_1 tumors.
ii. The grade of tumor is a second factor: there is a link
between stage and grade and 5 year survival rate is different.
iii. The tumor site also plays a role: the 5 year survival is
higher in tumors of the lateral walls than in those located at the
neck or the trigone.
iv. Of some importance are also the delay before first recurrence
and the number and volume of the tumors.

The Biological Potential

The most recent advance concerning the prognosis of a bladder
tumor is the description of many biological parameters of tumor
aggressiveness.

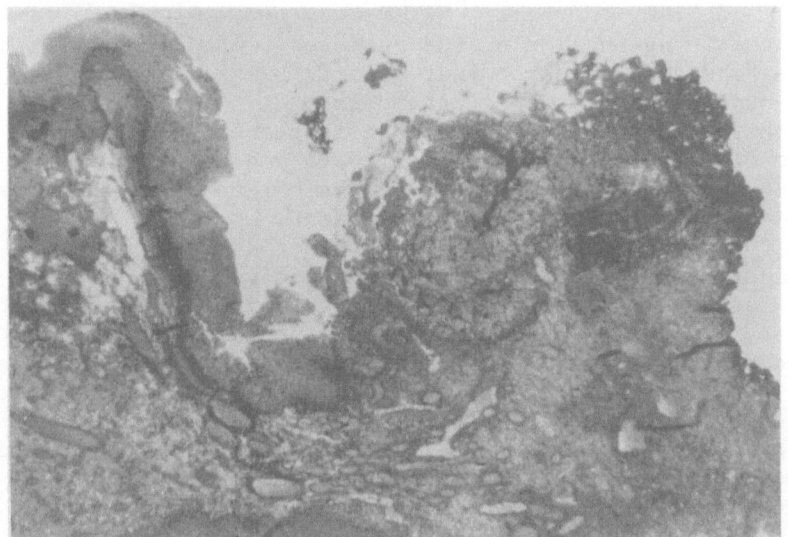

Fig. 5. A1 tumor: The chorion is only superficially invaded.

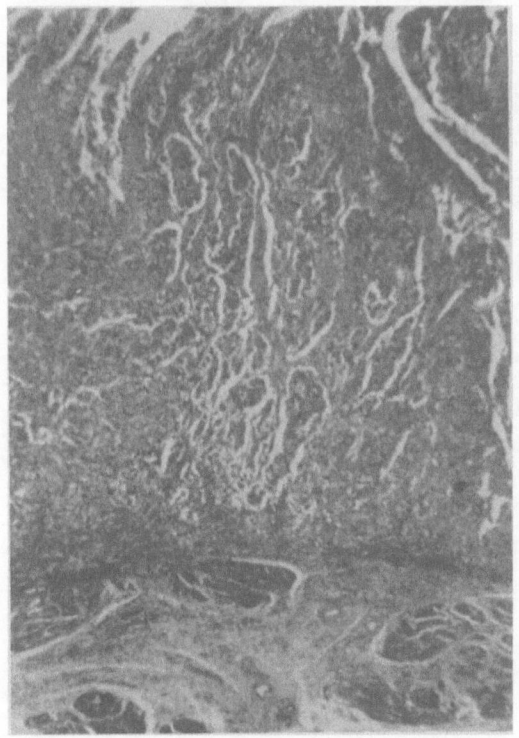

Fig. 6. A2 tumor: The chorion is totally invaded.

   i.   Cytogenetic evaluation of the resected tumor may be of some
value since "there is evidence that bladder tumors with high
chromosome numbers have a worse prognosis".
   ii.   The enzymatic approach seems more interesting as LDH is
elevated in bladder cancer and Bredin, Daly and Prout (4) have
demonstrated that the ratio of the various iso-enzymes of LDH is
different in high grade and low grade tumors.
iii.   Urinary carcino-embryonic antigen has also been studied but is
not sufficiently specific to be of prognostic value.
   iv.   The most important progress recently is in the immunological
approach.   A, B, H, cell surface antigens are normally present on
bladder mucosa and on some superficial tumors.   The loss of this
normal antigenic activity is correlated with the subsequent development of the invasive bladder cancer.   The antigenicity is assessed
by the specific red cell adherence test.   More recently, the test
has become more simple and much more reliable by using immunofluorescence to detect these antigens as demonstrated by three
French authors (5) (Fig. 7).

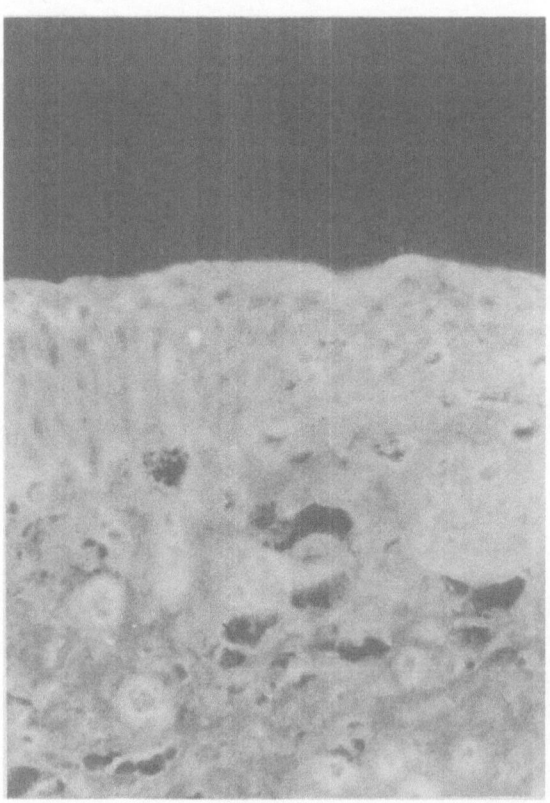

Fig. 7. Normal mucosa: the whole mucosa is fluorescent.

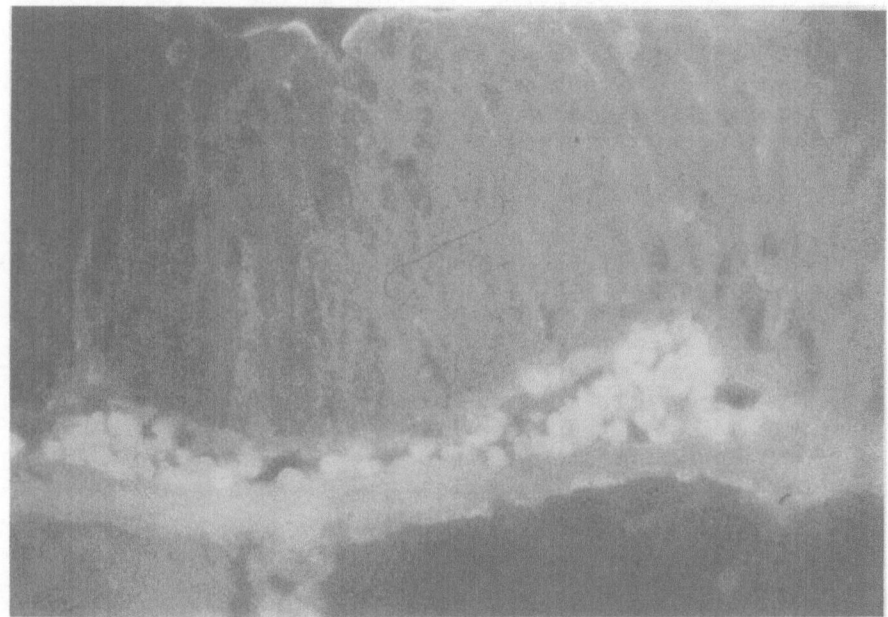

Fig. 8. "Negative" tumor: There is no fluorescence in the
urothelium. Fluorescence is limited to the red cells.

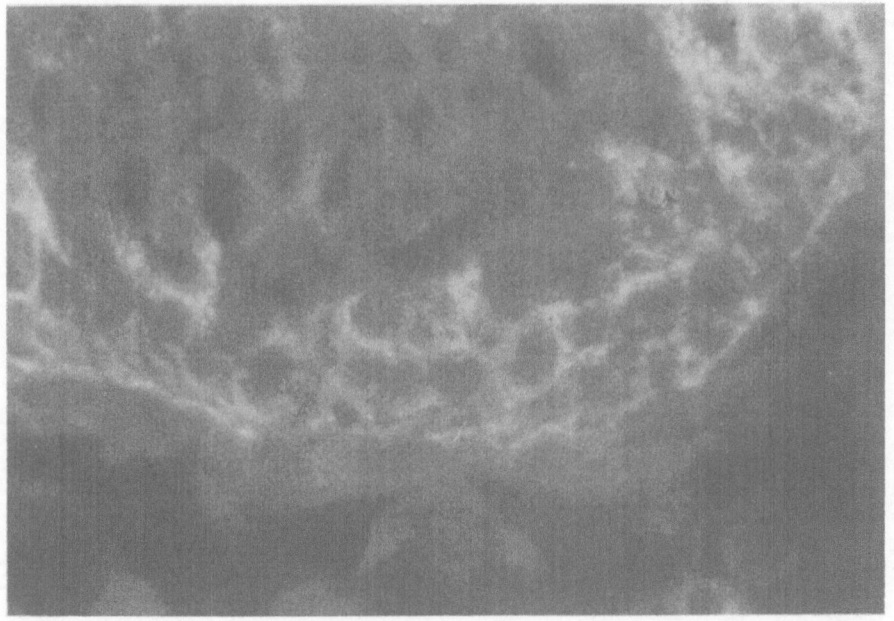

Fig. 9. Heterogeneous tumor.

When all the tumor is positive the whole mucosa is fluorescent; the red cells in the vessels are also positive. This is a homogeneous tumor and a good prognosis may be predicted. When the whole tumor is negative (Fig. 8) there is no fluorescence in the urothelium. Fluorescence is limited to the red cells and vascular walls. Here a bad prognosis is predicted. When the tumor is heterogenous (Fig. 9) fluorescence is lost in the superficial layers of the tumor but the deep layers remain fluorescent. Here the prognosis is intermediate as the tumor retains an "antigenic golden belt". The urothelial cells keep their developing polarity to the bladder lumen.

If the value of this biological approach is confirmed by larger studies it will open a new era in the treatment of superficial bladder tumors. For, if we have at our disposal such objective predictors of tumor invasion, the choice of the best treatment will in every case become easier, and we will be able to treat and hopefully to cure patients before invasion occurs. This possibility encourages me and allows me to end this paper on such a terrible disease with a note of hope.

REFERENCES

1. A. Steg and G. Allouch, Les facteurs de risque des tumeurs de vessie au Stade A. Description d'un nouveau parametre, Ann. Urol. 13: 215 (1979).
2. A. Steg, Le cancer de vessie in situ. A propos de 10 cas, Ann. Urol. 12: 73 (1978).
3. A.F. Althausen, G.R. Prout Jr., and J.J. Daly, Non papillary carcinoma of the bladder associated with cancer in situ, J. Urol. 116: 575 (1976).
4. H.C. Bredin, J.J. Daly, and G.R. Prout Jr., Lactic dehydrogenase isoenzymes in human bladder cancer, J. Urol. 113: 487 (1975).
5. C. Fella, J.C. Hammou, and J. Vacant, Les antigenes de surface ABH et l'antigene carcino-embryonnaire dans les tumeurs de vessie: leur mise en evidence par immunofluorescence, Ann. Urol. 14: 333 (1980).

STAGING OF BLADDER CANCER

M PAVONE-MACALUSO

University of Palermo
Palermo
Italy

INTRODUCTION

It is well established that the prognosis of cancer patients depends on several factors including:

- the local extension of the tumour, and the presence of single or multiple tumours;

- the presence or absence of lymph-node metastases and/or distant metastases;

- the presence or absence of neoplastic cells in lymphatics or in blood vessels;

- the histopathological type and architecture;

- the degree of cellular differentiation;

- the tumour - host relationship, including the patient's immunological reactivity.

These prognostic factors should be taken in consideration by the clinicians, if they wish to:

- give an indication of prognosis of a given patient;

- plan the most appropriate treatment for the same patient and, in a more extended field, if they wish to compare their own results with those of other investigators.

The practice of dividing cancer cases into groups, the so-called "stages" arose from the fact that survival and recovery rates are higher for patients in whom the disease is localized, than for those in whom the disease has extended beyond the site of origin. The term "grading" refers to the cellular differentiation and degree of anaplasia.

The need for a classification of cancer is of paramount importance, especially to facilitate the exchange of information between treatment centres and to contribute to the continuing investigation of human cancer.

Any classification should be based on a rigid definition of each term, as confusion and misunderstanding are liable to arise when people attempt to communicate using different languages. More commonly, however, confusion arises between two people using the same language, each attaching a different meaning to what appears to be a common term.

The U.I.C.C. has proposed the TNM classification, in order to reach agreement on the recording of accurate information on the extent of the disease for each anatomical site. The TNM classification is gaining world-wide acceptance. It has been adopted, for urological tumours, by the WHO and by the EORTC, as well as by some leading American and Japanese groups. At a recent WHO meeting on bladder cancer, it was strongly advocated that whilst alternative classifications might still be used, the TNM classification should also be given, as a universal code.

The TNM classification can be defined as a kind of short-hand notation, where T represents the extent of the primary tumour, N the condition of the regional lymph nodes and M the presence or absence of distant metastases.

The first TNM classification of bladder tumours was presented in 1974 and subsequently revised in 1978. The present classification, introduced in January 1979, is intended to remain unchanged for at least 10 years, unless some major advances make modifications unavoidable. The differences between the original and the present classifications are not very great. New terms have been introduced, including Ta for the bladder and the symbols pT, pN, pM, y and r, as well as the C category, which apply to tumours of all sites.

ASSESSMENT OF THE PRIMARY TUMOUR

It should be stressed that the T category is a "pre-treatment classification" indicating local spread only by clinical assessment. In bladder cancer, the minimum requirements for the assessment of T-category are as follows:

- Clinical examination;
- Urography;
- Cystoscopy;
- Bimanual examination under anesthesia;
- Biopsy or transurethral resection of the tumour (if indicated)
  prior to definitive treatment.

The local infiltration can be assessed again, after the
treatment. If the treatment is surgery, the "post-surgical histopathological classification" will be applied. This was expressed
with the symbol P in the 1974 TNM classification. Since 1978, its
denomination is pT. Similarly, if the assessment of regional lymph-
nodes and distant metastases is based on surgical specimens, the
corresponding symbols are pN and pM respectively. Figure 1 depicts
the local extent categories for bladder tumours according to the
1978 TNM classification.

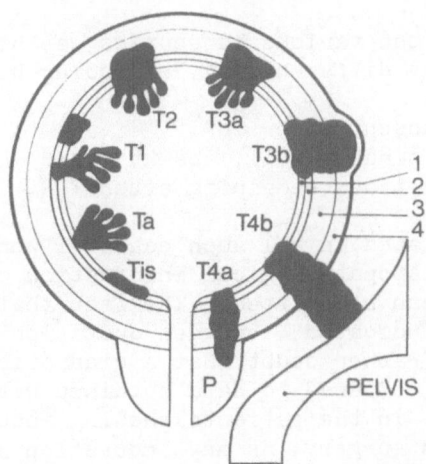

Fig. 1. T categories, according to the 1978 TNM classification.
         1. Urothelium. 2. Submucosa. 3. Muscle. 4. Serosa.

The 1978 guidebook defines such categories as follows:

To = no evidence of primary tumour.
Tis= flat carcinoma in situ.
Ta = papillary carcinoma, not invading the lamina propria.
T1 = invasion of the lamina propria.
T2 = invasion of the superficial muscle.
T3a= invasion of deep muscle.
T3b= invasion through the bladder wall.
T4 = tumour extending to neighbouring strucutres.
T4a= infiltration of prostate, uterus or vagina.
T4b= fixation to the pelvic and/or abdominal wall.
Tx = the minimum requirements to assess the primary tumour
     cannot be met.

The suffix (m) may be added to the appropriate T category
to indicate multiple tumours, e.g. T1 (m).

There are a few comments to be made about this classification.
It is clearly stated that there should be histological or
cytological verification of the disease. Biopsy or TUR,
prior to definitive treatment, are listed among the investigations
necessary for a minimum assessment, but only "if indicated".
Therefore, the various categories can be applied even without
a biopsy, but only on the basis of cytology and bimanual
palpation before and after complete TUR of the lesion, for tumours
from T1 to T3.

The definition of the various categories can be given,
therefore, in a slightly different way, excluding biopsy reports:

T1: mobile mass, absent after TUR.
T2: induration of bladder wall, absent after TUR.
T3: mass and induration, remaining after TUR.

As TUR is contemplated in all such cases, I wonder why it
is accepted that the histopathological information obtained from
the resected material can be omitted. The fact that TUR-biopsy is
a requirment only "if indicated", between quotation marks, leaves
me rather puzzled as I rather doubt that a classification based on
biopsy evidence can be compared to data obtained without it. This
is certainly impossible in the patients showing recurrence after
irradiation or previous surgery, as any induration of the bladder
wall will be of doubtful significance.

Papilloma is excluded from this classification, which is by
definition, a classification of malignant tumours, whereas it was
accepted in the previous one, of 1974, classified under TO. In
the present instructions a rather confusing sentence reads:
Papilloma is excluded, but such cases should be listed under

the category Ta. Category Ta is defined as "papillary non-invasive carcinoma". It seems obvious that, if Ta is a carcinoma by definition, it cannot include papilloma. In my view, papilloma should be excluded altogether.

To return to the question of biopsy, it can probably be omitted only in the unequivocal T4 lesion, if positive cytology is available; I do not think it can be omitted in the Tis and in the Ta tumours. It is also impossible to distinguish between a papilloma and a Ta transitional cell carcinoma on the one hand, and between a Ta and a T1 tumour on the other, without a TUR-biopsy. Diathermy does not allow a proper T classification. Furthermore, although a diagnosis of ca in situ is warranted on merely cytological grounds, the location and the multiplicity of the lesions can only be given by multiple biopsies.

If a biopsy is requested in all cases (except perhaps in the T4) and if a complete removal of the lesion by TUR is contemplated in T1, T2 and early T3 lesions, biopsy and definitive treatment will be coincident in most Ta, T1 and at least some T2 cases. Should we then classify these cases under the T or the pT category?

This is a rather controversial point and the attitude of different groups is not uniform. In the introduction to the TNM booklet, it states that the T, or pre-treatment clinical classification, "may be based, in some instances, on the evidence derived from surgical exploration prior to decision as to definitive treatment". I think that this is the case in papillary bladder tumour, as the decision whether the TUR performed does or does not represent the definitive treatment, is usually taken after and not before the pathologist's report. Only in the case of small, superficial papillary tumours, where TUR appears to be, a priori, the definitive treatment, it is perhaps justified to classify such tumours under the pT rather than under the T category.

Coming back to the 1978 classification, the new symbol Ta has been introduced. As this will last for at least another 10 years, we can only accept it without discussion.

I agree that it is important to distinguish between tumours invading or not invading the lamina propria, as they have a different prognosis. This has been clearly shown by Rübben et al. (6) in 1980, and it is strange that this had not been recognized earlier. The trouble is that what we now call T1 is different from that which we called T1 before 1978. This is likely to create confusion. Why did they not baptise these two conditions T1a and T1b instead of introducing this unusual code Ta, which does not exist in any other site in oncological nomenclature? However, it is too late for recriminations.

ASSESSMENT OF THE NODES

The N categories have remained unchanged. The regional lymph
nodes are defined as the pelvic nodes below the bifurcation of the
common iliac arteries, whereas the juxta-regional nodes are the
inguinal nodes, the common iliac nodes and the para-aortic nodes.
Let me recall briefly:

No = no regional node involvement.
N1 = single homolateral regional node involved.
N2 = contra - or bilateral or multiple regional nodes.
N3 = fixed regional mass. Free space between mass and
     primary tumour.
N4 = juxta-regional nodes.

It should be remembered that if metastases are found in
lymph nodes beyond the regional and the juxta-regional stations,
this is classified as M1, for it is considered equivalent to a
distant metastasis.

The minimum requirements for assessment of the N category are:
clinical examination, lymphography and urography. Unfortunately,
this does not enable us to make a valuable assessment of the N
category, since lymphography is so unreliable that many people
strongly feel that it is not justified as a routine investigation.
Therefore, most patients will fall into the Nx category, since the
minimum defined requirement has not been met. The present rules
do not take into consideration echography, CT scan or staging
lymphadenectomy. However,it is desirable that they are employed,
when available and indicated, provided that their use is recorded.
In this context, the new C-factor can be usefully applied.

C-factor or "level of certainty" is an optional, flexible
system for indicating the information on which the classification
is based.

The C-factor category definition is as follows:

C1 = evidence from clinical examination only.
C2 = evidence obtained by special diagnostic means
     (CT scan and echography obviously apply to this group).
C3 = evidence from surgical exploration only (the so-called
     surgical staging).
C4 = evidence from definitive surgery including the complete
     examination of the therapeutically resected specimen.
     This corresponds to the pN classification with regard
     to lymph nodes.
C5 = evidence from autopsy.

Can we therefore classify our cases as, for example, N2 C2 or N1 C3, even without lymphangiography? I think that we can but it is not clearly stated in the TNM rules.

One last point about the nodes. The information obtained from surgical staging was expressed, prior to 1979, as N- or N+ respectively for nodes with or without microscopic evidence of metastasis. This was added to the clinical category. Now it will be substituted by the pN categories: pNO, pNl, etc.

ASSESSMENT OF METASTASES

The 1978 classification for the M categories is different from the older one, in that Mla, b, c and d are no longer recommended. There is only one category - M1, indicating evidence of distant metastases, irrespective of their number, location or extension. Mo implies no evidence of metastases and Mx indicates that the minimum requirements to assess the presence of distant metastases cannot be met. pM categories correspond to the M categories. pM represents the evidence based on post-surgical histopathologic examination, while M is only based on clinical evidence, including physical examination and radiography. Isotope studies are recommended, when indicated, but are not essential for the clinical M classification. Again, the C-factor can be added: e.g. C2, evidence from special diagnostic means.

HISTOPATHOLOGICAL ASSESSMENT

The histopathological categories, with regard to the bladder, conform to the classification recommended in 1973 by the World Health Organization.

The G grading, from G1 to G3 and the L-categories which related to the invasion of lymphatics, remain unchanged.

Let me recall briefly both headings:

G1 = Well differentiated.
G2 = Medium degree of differentiation.
G3 = Poorly differentiated or undifferentiated.
Gx = Grade cannot be assessed.

LO = No lymphatic invasion within the bladder wall.
L1 = Evidence of invasion of superficial lyphatics.
L2 = Evidence of invasion of deep lymphatics.
Lx = Lymphatic invasion cannot be assessed.

The 1978 TNM classification introduces two new symbols: y symbol: this applies to cases where definitive surgery

is performed after treatment by other methods,
such as radiotherapy. Example: ypT2, pN1, M0.
These cases must be reported separately.
   r symbol: this indicates recurrent tumours. Example: rT1,
             Nx, M0. This should be widely applied in the case
             of bladder tumours.

CONCLUSIONS

The TNM classification is a dual system - clinical and post-
surgical. The clinical classification is less accurate but is more
important for the purposes of reporting and evaluation, especially
for comparison between surgical treatment and irradiation or
chemotherapy. It is important to emphasize that the clinical TNM
categories, once established must remain unchanged. Stage grouping,
for bladder tumours is not recommended at present.

This last statement may give rise to some discussion. Some
people, especially in USA, feel that the TNM classification, although
more descriptive and detailed, is in fact too complicated. These
workers still prefer, for practical purposes, the original classification by Jewett-Strong (3) in 1946 with or without the more
recent modifications advocated by Marshall in 1952 and by Olsson
and de Vere White (4) in 1979.

We are supporters of the TNM classification, not only as a
matter of discipline, as we believe it is right to adhere to an
international agreement, but also for the many advantages it offers.

Probably its most important advantage lies in the distinction
between clinical and post-surgical categories, enabling comparison
between treatments, whereas no comparison is possible when the same
stage can be applied to clinical and surgical material.

A tumour classification must be useful for the clinician,
whether he be surgeon, radiotherapist or chemotherapist. It should
not depend on surgical extirpation as the behaviour of a tumour and
its reaction to non-surgical methods of treatment cannot be evaluated
if the classification is only valid for operative specimens.

Information obtained at operation is not generally admissible
for clinical classification, but may be used as an addition to it.
I recall that the symbol pT, formerly P, from 1 to 4, refers to the
depth of infiltration of the tumour within an organ or tissue, as
assessed on the operative specimen.

Any classification is valid only if it has practical significance, and is accurate and reproducible. Unfortunately, the
clinical staging for bladder tumour is reliable only in part.
Not only is lymphangiography quite unreliable, but also clinical

T staging is not very accurate. As the degree of penetration of
the bladder wall increases, our ability to assess the infiltration
accurately decreases. The correlation between clinical and
surgical-pathological staging is 80-90% in Ta and T1, but falls to
50-70% in the higher stages.

Understaging is more likely than overstaging in the higher
stage tumours. The differentiation between superficial and deep
muscle infiltration, i.e. T2 - T3a or B1 - B2 is particularly
difficult. Even the practical value of such a distinction has
been questioned. Many series, following Jewett's (2) first claim,
indicate that the 5 year survival is much worse if the deeper muscle
is invaded. However, during the past few years, several authors
have expressed their doubts about the practical value of T2 - T3
subdivision in determining prognosis and treatment alternatives.
Richie et al. (5) from UCLA reported a 40% 5 year survival rate
after preoperative radiation and cystectomy whether muscular
invasion was superficial or deep. Also in Whitmore's experience (8)
the depth of muscular infiltration did not affect the survival rate
in patients treated with cystectomy plus preoperative irradiation.

However, if cystectomy only was performed 5 year survival in
T2 patients was 60%, compared with 25% for T3a. A recent report by
Bredael et al. (1), supports the concept that at least in patients
treated by surgery alone, the prognosis is adversely affected by
the depth of muscular penetration, as assessed by the conventional
methods of clinical staging. Therefore, in reply to the provocative
question by Jewett: two-B or not two-B?, the answer is that in spite
of a high degree of inaccuracy, the differentiation between B1 and
B2 or T3a, still should be maintained.

In spite of such shortcomings accurate staging is essential
in any evaluation of a bladder tumour and we fully agree with
Olsson's conclusion (4) that the extent of spread - or stage - of
the bladder cancer still remains the single most important factor
affecting prognosis.

REFERENCES

1. J.J. Croker, B.P. Croker, and J.F. Glenn, Curability of
    Invasive Bladder Cancer Treated by Radical Cystectomy,
    Eur. Urol. 6: 206-210 (1980).
2. H.J. Jewett, Carcinoma of the Bladder. Influence of Depth of
    Infiltration on the 5-year Results Following Complete Extirpation
    of the Primary Growth, J. Urol. 67: 672-676 (1952).
3. H.J. Jewett and G.H. Strong, Infiltrating Carcinoma of the
    Bladder. Relation of Depth of Penetration of the Bladder Wall
    to Incidence of Local Extension and Metastases, J. Urol. 55:
    366-372 (1946).

4. C.A. Olsson and R.W. de Vere White, Cancer of the Bladder, in:
    "Principles and Management of Urologic Cancer," N. Javadpour, ed,
    William and Wilkins Co., Baltimore, pp 337-376 (1979).
5. J.P. Richie, D.G. Skinner, and J.J. Kaufman, Radical Cystectomy
    for Carcinoma of the Bladder. 16 Years of Experience, J.Urol.
    113: 186-189 (1975).
6. H. Rübben, H.H. Dahm, J. Bubenzer, and W. Lutzeyer, TNM
    Classification of Urinary Bladder Tumours: Value of Ta Category
    for Non Infiltrating Exophytic Tumour, in: "Bladder Tumours and
    Other Topics in Urological Oncology," M. Pavone-Macaluso,
    P.H. Smith, and F. Edsmyr, eds., Plenum Press, London and
    New York, pp 9-12 (1980).
7. U.I.C.C.: TNM Classification of Malignant Tumours, Geneva, 1978.
8. W.F. Whitmore Jr, M.A. Batata, M.A. Ghoneim, H. Grabstald, and
    A. Unal, Radical Cystectomy with or without Prior Irradiation
    in the Treatment of Bladder Cancer, J. Urol. 118: 184-187 (1977).

TRANSURETHRAL ULTRASONOGRAPHY - BLADDER CANCER STAGING AND OTHER

CLINICAL APPLICATION

T NIIJIMA AND S NAKAMURA

Department of Urology
University of Tokyo
Japan

INTRODUCTION

The newly developed technique of transurethral ultrasonography
makes it possible to see a cross sectional image of the bladder.
This is useful in bladder cancer staging and has some other clinical
applications such as in the follow up study of bladder cancer.
Observing the bladder wall, accurate diagnostic information of
cancer staging can be obtained preoperatively as if we were examining
a surgical specimen of the tumor.

In the past, several diagnostic methods have been developed to
examine the infiltration of the bladder wall by cancer - cystoscopy
and bimanual examination under anaesthesia, radiological techniques
including cystography and pelvic angiography, and the recently
developed diagnostic techniques of X-ray computed tomography and
ultrasonotomography which are the only two ways of obtaining a
cross sectional image of the bladder.

By CT scanning cross sections of the tumor, the bladder and
other pelvic organs are visualized clearly. However, the shape of
the tumor base is not well defined, because the absorption coef-
ficient of the X-ray is almost the same in both the tumor and the
bladder wall. Clear observation of the tumor base is difficult even
with enhancement of the tumor by contrast media.

Ultrasonic scanning via the abdominal wall (1,4,7) has a similar
disadvantage in that the fine structure of the tumor and the bladder
wall is difficult to visualise. Although transrectal scanning (2)
brings the transducer closer to the bladder, the ultimate image is

not satisfactory. To visualise the bladder wall clearly, it is
important for the beam to hit the wall perpendicularly.

     In the transurethral radial scanning system (5) the transducer
is placed in the bladder. The bladder wall can be scanned by a
probe inside the bladder and the sonic beam radiated from this
probe hits the wall perpendicularly. Then, a clear cross sectional
image of the bladder wall is obtained in almost its whole area. The
prostate may also be scanned (3).

     However even with this prototype transurethral scanning probe
it was difficult to obtain a clear image of the wall in the dome or
at the neck of the bladder because the reflected beam of ultrasound
from these sites in the bladder is not easily caught by the transducer. We resolved this problem by developing a probe with a head
angulating device (Fig. 1). The cross section of the dome can be
obtained by transmitting in an upward direction, and the bladder
neck image by transmitting in a downward direction.

     This system has been used for bladder cancer staging and the
authors have reported tomograms of various stages, interpretation
of the tomograms for cancer staging, and clinical results in twenty
tumors (6).

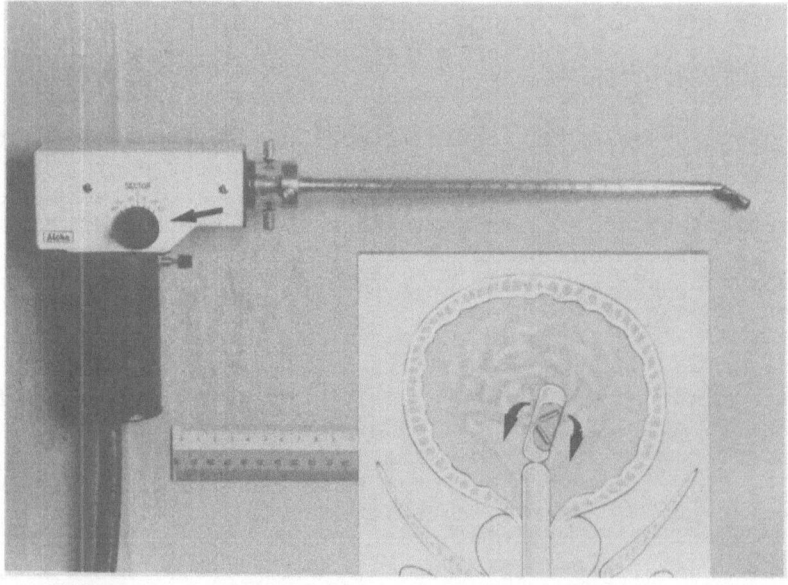

Fig. 1. Transurethral intravesical scanner with a head angulating
         device. The head may be bent freely up to 45 degrees to
         either side by a dial (arrow). Two transducers are placed
         facing each other at 90 degrees, to radiate the sonic beam
         in any direction.

METHOD AND RESULTS

The scanning procedure is quite simple. At first, the outer sheath of the probe is introduced into the bladder with the obturator. Then the probe itself is introduced into the bladder. The bladder is filled with water. Watching the real-time image on the CRT monitor, the angle of the probe is adjusted to obtain the best view of the bladder.

Tomograms of the bladder at various levels are shown on Fig. 2. At first, a cross section of a portion of the dome is obtained (Fig. 2a). Then, a larger cross section of the corpus of the bladder is visualised. Outside the bladder, the external iliac vessels and hydro-ureter are also observed on the tomogram (Fig. 2b). Where the bladder is distended with water, its contour is deformed by the os ischii. Superficial cancer is observed, in this case (Fig. 2c). The os pubis may be seen anterior to the bladder (Fig. 2d). The head angulating device is especially effective for the observation of the bladder wall near the neck. Trigonal elevation and the bladder wall close to the neck are shown on Fig. 2e and 2f.

The transurethral intravesical scanning system enables clear observation of the tumor and of the bladder wall. Since images of the tumor, mucosal oedema and the muscle layers of the bladder are differentiated from each other, the diagnostic criteria used in pathological staging may be easily determined from the sonogram (Table 1).

TABLE 1

DIAGNOSTIC CRITERIA OF BLADDER CANCER STAGING BY

TRANSURETHRAL ULTRASONOGRAPHY

Ta, T1   Image of muscle layer is intact at tumor base

T2   Image of muscle layer is superficially indented
             at tumor base

T3   Image of muscle layer is deeply indented or has
             disappeared at tumor base

T4   The prostatic image is deformed or the tomogram
             shows some other perivesical structure is
             involved in tumor extension

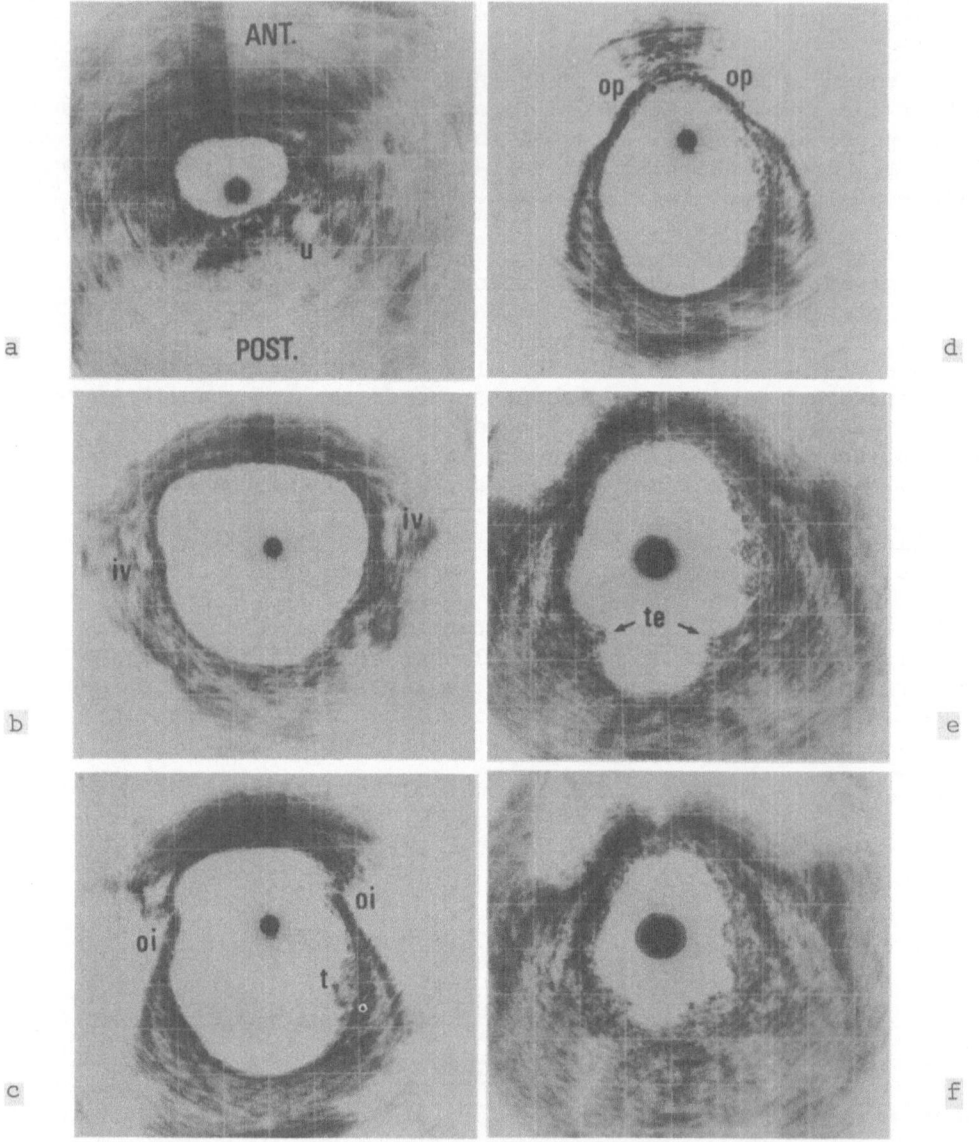

Fig. 2. Tomograms of the bladder at various levels.
    a. Tomogram of bladder at the dome, Cross-section of hydro-
       ureter (u) is observed.
    b. Iliac vessels (iv) outside the bladder.
    c. Bladder is deformed by os ischii (oi), superficial tumor (t)
       on left lateral wall.
    d. Os pubis (op) anterior to the bladder.
    e. Trigonal elevations (te).
    f. Tomogram of bladder close to the neck.
(Magnification in Figs. e and f is twice that of the others)

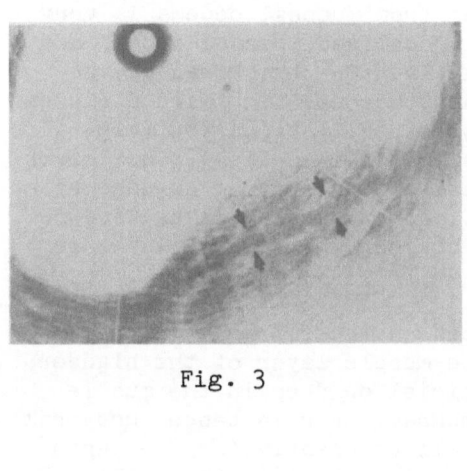

Fig. 3

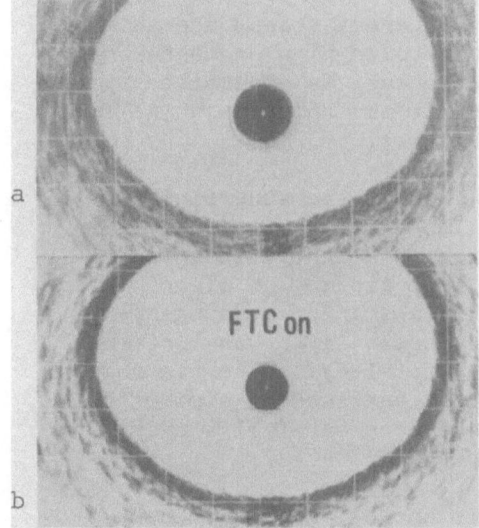

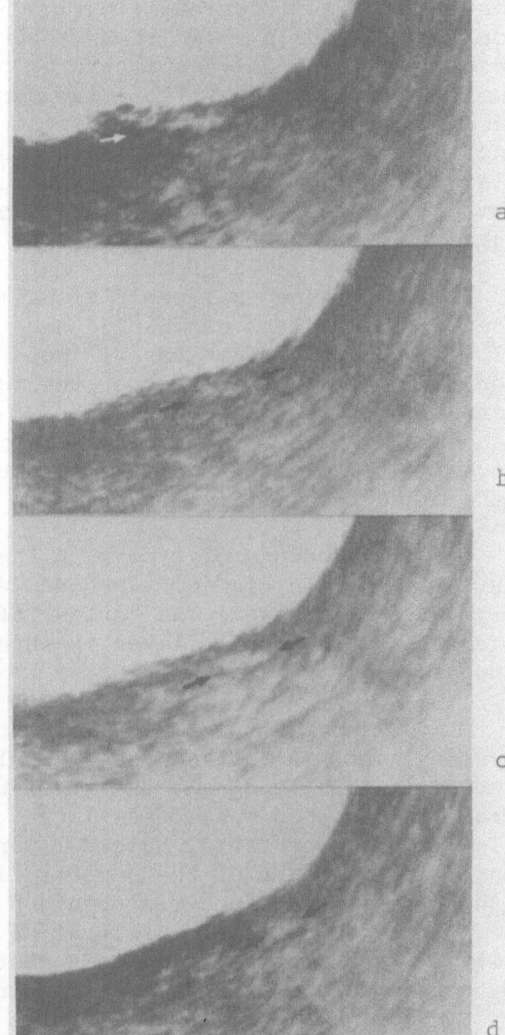

Fig. 4   Fig. 5

Fig. 3.   Tomogram of localised mucosal oedema and underlying muscle
           layer (arrows).
Fig. 4.   Effect of F.T.C. circuit. a. and b. are at the same site in
           the bladder. b. is displayed under F.T.C. circuit adjust-
           ment and the circumference of the wall is emphasised.
Fig. 5.   Tomogram of ureteral penetration of the wall. Ureter out-
           side the bladder (d). Ureter is deep (c), intermediate
           (b) and superficial (a) in the bladder wall.

The differentiation of muscle layer from mucosal oedema is very important in tumor staging. In Fig. 3, localised mucosal oedema and underlying muscle layer is shown separately. The thickness of the bladder wall is roughly estimated on the tomogram. The circumference of wall is emphasized by fast time constant (FTC) circuitry (Fig. 4). Although ultrasound can detect slight submucosal swelling, this layer is not always visualised. In such cases, cancer staging is done by neglecting the thickness of the mucosal and submucosal layer, and assuming that the muscle layer and the bladder wall are the same in thickness.

The tumor base is clearly visualised on the tomogram, since cancer tissue is less echogenic than the muscle layer of the bladder wall. Whether the tumor base is superficial or deep in the muscle layer is directly determined on the tomogram. For instance, ureteral penetration of the bladder wall is visualised clearly and the depth of the ureter is determined on the tomogram. At first the ureter is outside the bladder and is then deep, intermediate and superficial in the bladder wall (Fig. 5).

Typical findings of tumors in the different stages are shown in Figs. 6 and 9. In Fig. 6, a pedunculated tumor with no muscular infiltration is shown. The contour of the wall is emphasised by the FTC circuit. The muscle layer is intact at the tumor base (no image of mucosal oedema is seen in these tomograms).

Fig. 7 shows a tumor with infiltration in the superficial muscular layer. Although a submucosal image (little arrows) is observed in this tomogram, the tumor base is slightly indented (arrow) beyond this submucosal image. This finding of slight indentation in the superficial muscle layer is a sign of a category T2 tumor. Infiltration of the superficial muscle layer was confirmed by the pathological specimen obtained by total cystectomy in this case. Since superficial infiltration is visualised as a minor deformity on the tomogram, diagnosis must be done carefully, examining many sequential tomograms at narrow intervals.

In Fig. 8, deeply invasive tumor is shown. Mucosal oedema (little arrows) is also observed in this case. Thickening of the muscular layer is evident at the lateral margin of the tumor and tumor penetration of the wall was observed on the tomogram. After total cystectomy, infiltration beyond the bladder wall was confirmed pathologically.

Diagnosis of distant metastasis by intravesical scanning is of course impossible. However, pelvic organs such as the seminal vesicles and uterus are visualised. The prostate is displayed clearly by radical scanning at the level of the prostatic urethra. If the tomogram shows infiltration of the prostate or other perivesical structure, the diagnosis of category T4 is possible. Fig. 9

a

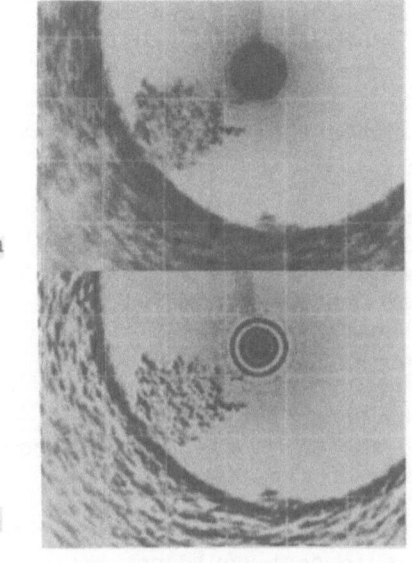

b

Fig. 6

a

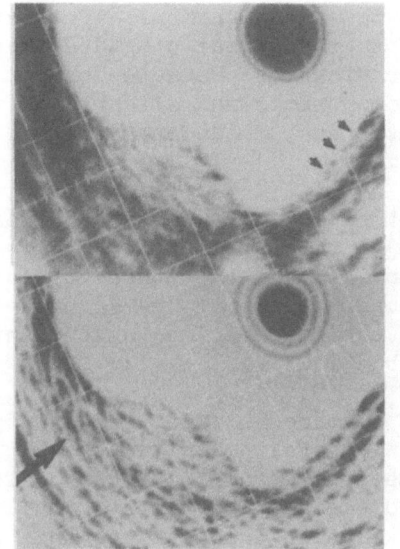

b

Fig. 8

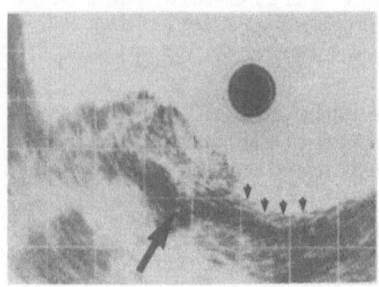

Fig. 7

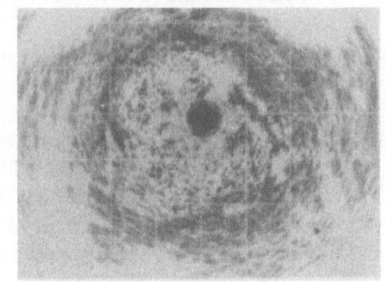

Fig. 9

Fig. 6. Tomogram of a pedunculated tumor with no muscular infilt-
        ration (pT1). b. displayed under F.T.C. circuit adjustment.
        Image of muscle layer is intact at the tumor base.

Fig. 7. Tomogram of a tumor with superficial muscular infiltration
        (T2). Little arrows indicate slight mucosal oedema. Image
        of muscle layer is slightly indented at tumor base (arrow).

Fig. 8. Tomogram of a deeply infiltrative tumor (T3). a. little
        arrows indicate mucosal oedema. b. thickening of the muscle
        layer at the tumor margin (arrow) and tumor penetration of
        the wall are observed.

Fig. 9. Tomogram of a prostate with bladder cancer infiltration.
        The contour of the prostate is irregularly swollen but
        internal echos have a rather homogeneus pattern.

demonstrates a tomogram of a prostate infiltrated by bladder cancer.
Compared to the normal prostate image thus scanned, the irregularly
swollen contour is characteristic. The internal echo pattern is
rather homogeneous and slightly different even from prostatic cancer,
which often has a nodular pattern in its circumferential and internal
echo image.

In the past two years, 64 cases of bladder cancer have been
examined by this transurethral intravesical scanning (25 cases were
treated by TUR and the others by open operation). Of those treated
by open operation, tomograms in 24 cases were compared carefully
with the excised specimen which contained the full thickness of the
wall (Table 2).

The ultrasonic findings corresponded to the pathological stage,
except in the following two cases. In one case which was over-staged,
an intense reflection caused by calcification on the tumor surface
disturbed clear tumor observation. Down staging by preoperative
therapy was also suspected in this case. In an under-staged case,
cellular infiltration in the superficial muscle coat could not be
determined on the tomogram.

In 25 cases treated by TUR, no muscular infiltration was observed
on the tomograms. The pathological findings and the clinical course
after operation were compatible with the preoperative diagnosis.

The accuracy of cancer staging by transurethral intravesical
scanning is very high when compared to ordinary diagnostic methods.
It has been stressed that the staging of bladder cancer is important,
since it determines the mode of treatment. But is was quite unsatisfactory that exact staging could only be determined from pathological
examination of the specimen excised at operation. This problem may

TABLE 2

ULTRASONIC FINDINGS AND PATHOLOGICAL STAGING IN CASES
EXAMINED IN WHICH THE EXCISED SPECIMEN CONTAINED THE
FULL THICKENSS OF THE WALL

		pT1	pT2	pT3	Total
	Ta,T1	11	1	0	12
Ultrasonic Findings	T2	0	3	0	3
	T3	1	0	8	9
	Total	12	4	8	24

be solved by this scanning method, since it allows preoperative staging which is as accurate as pathological examination. It is also useful for the observation of tumor image under treatment.

The procedure of transurethral resection of bladder tumor can be monitored by transurethral endoscopic scanning. A scanner, equipped with an adapter, and the resectoscope are interchangeably attached to the resectoscope sheath. Monitoring the procedure by ultrasound, the operator can know how deep and to what extend the tumor must be resected.

Reduction in tumor size by radio-chemotherapy has also been followed up by ultrasonography in a case of malignant lymphoma of the bladder. A large deeply infiltrating tumor became smaller and flatter after radiotherapy and, following chemotherapy, the tumor disappeared; the bladder wall was almost normal five months later.

This endoscopic scanning method by intravesically intubated probe is useful for observation of tumor image, and for accurate cancer staging as well as monitoring under various types of therapy. The scanning procedure is simple and important diagnostic information can be obtained which would otherwise be unobtainable.

(The tomograms shown in this presentation have been obtained by using various transurethral scanners developed in our clinic.)

REFERENCES

1. E. Barnett and P. Morley, Ultrasound in the investigation of space-occupying lesions of the urinary tract, Brit. J. Radiol. 44: 733 (1971).
2. K. Harada, D. Igari, Y. Tanahashi, H. Watanabe, M. Saitoh, and T. Mishina, Staging of bladder tumors by means of transrectal ultrasonography, J. Clin. Ultrasound 5: 388 (1977).
3. H.H. Holm and A. Northeved, A transurethral ultrasonic scanner, J. Urol. 111: 238 (1974).
4. I.S. McLaughlin, P. Morley, R.F. Deane, E. Barnett, A.G. Graham, and K.F. Kyle, Ultrasound in the staging of bladder tumors, Brit. J. Urol. 47: 51 (1975).
5. L.I. Micsky, Gynecologic ultrasonography, Diagnostic ultrasound, D.L. King, ed., The C.V. Mosby Company, Saint Louis, 207 (1974).
6. S. Nakamura and T. Niijima, Staging of bladder cancer by ultrasonography: a new technique by transurethral intravesical scanning, J. Urol. (in press)
7. T. Shiraishi, Ultrasonic diagnosis for urinary tract - mainly for determination of staging of bladder tumor, Jap. J. Urol. 69: 47 (1978).

THERAPEUTIC APPROACHES

CHAIRMAN'S SUMMARY

F EDSMYR
Radiumhemmet, Stockholm
Sweden

The development of new methods of treatment in patients suffering from urinary bladder cancer has been going on for almost three decades. There is always the therapeutic problem of knowing which form of therapy is best for the different stages and grades. At the WHO Collaborating Centre for urinary bladder cancer in Stockholm, the poorly malignant, exophytic, non-palpable urinary bladder tumors have been treated surgically for many years. Full irradiation has been given to the advanced, palpable and fixed tumors - T3-T4. The middle group of highly malignant, exophytic, non-palpable tumors has been treated for the last 10 years by preoperative irradiation followed by cystectomy. The results of treatment are better than those from surgery or external irradiation alone. Studies by Whitmore in the United States and Van der Werf-Messing in the Netherlands of selected patients with T3 tumors have shown similar results.

The results reported by Professor Van der Werf-Messing on the use of radium implantation for tumors less than 5 cm in size are encouraging and this form of therapy seems to make an alternative to the other established methods of treatment. Other radioactive isotopes have been used in the United States for tumor implantation into the urinary bladder.

However, there is a clear need for improved methods of treatment especially of the more advanced tumors of categories T3-T4. In Stockholm, external irradiation has been given to these groups of patients since 1957. Within the last few years treatment has been randomized between either Bestatin, an immunostimulating drug, or no additional therapy after the irradiation. For some time a new method of radiotherapy has been used in which treatment is given three times daily - super fractionation - as compared with one treatment daily. On evaluation of the five year results, there is a significant improvement in survival at one and two years for the superfractionated patients who also showed a significantly higher incidence of patients who were tumor free. However, these differences levelled out later and, at five years, the survival is equal in the superfractionated patients and in the control group.

We have to find a method making use of any improvement in results which appears. It may be possible to use chemotherapy combined with, or following, irradiation and scientific, randomized studies are needed to determine the value, if any, of such therapy.

DYNAMIC EVALUATION OF BLADDER CANCER

G R PROUT Jr.

Department of Surgery
Massachusetts General Hospital
Boston, U.S.A.

Previous papers have been published which deal with some of the material which follows (1, 2, 3). Because bladder cancer is so heterogenous, it becomes essential that one characterize and classify each patient as carefully as possible. As can be shown, the multifactorial elements of bladder cancer in a given patient or group of patients may have more influence on the outcome of therapy than the therapy itself.

Jewett and Strong (4) and later, Marshall (5), directed the attention of two generations of Urologists to the relationship of invasion to nodal metastases. Schematic representation of the staging schema (Fig. 1) was in keeping with the times and provided for a reasonable means of communication. It embodied bimanual examination (a help, if positive) and transurethral resection of the tumor. Scarcely anyone collected the fragments in three bottles; rather, deep bites were taken. These were often charily obtained and charred as well - a matter of great importance to the Pathologist who was then required to provide information on cell type, grade, depth of muscle invasion and involvement of lymphatics. The system left much to be desired and omitted several important items. Carcinoma-in-situ had just been described by Melicow (1952) when staging reached its full development. There was and remains no place for TIS in the O-D$_2$ system. Some of the other problems, not all solvable by any technique, are listed below.

1. There is no certain way to determine whether the staging is clinical or pathological.
2. There is no way to indicate multiplicity of lesions.
3. When the lesion is metastatic there is no way to learn about the primary tumor.

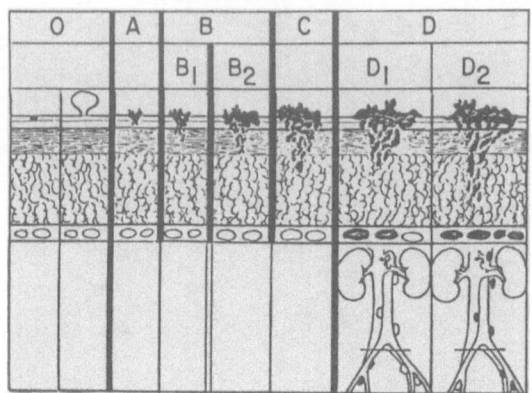

Fig. 1.   Jewett, Strong and Marshall system of staging bladder
          carcinoma

4.   No systematic plan for providing grade is included.
5.   There is no provision for indicating the morphology of the
     primary tumor, i.e., sessile, papillary or solid.

     In spite of these shortcomings, American Urologists seem to
prefer the O-D$_2$ system to the TNM system of the UICC. This latter
system was introduced to the United States some twenty years ago,
but the Urological community felt uncomfortable with it. At least,
no advantage was perceived and the UICC system was eschewed. As an
afterthought it may be that the lack of the requirement of histological confirmation of tissue penetration may have dimmed some
Urologists' enthusiasm. The Urological community had just emerged
from a long bout of polemics regarding this point and the UICC
"and/or" in T staging may have been the cause of rejection. Currently, we are working to improve the American Joint Committee's
classification which is receiving wider and wider acceptance. We
do feel that precision is very important, and so we have formed an
additional category of tumor, those that are carcinomas, not
papillomas, but papillary in configuration, and are confined to the
mucosa. These we have entitled "Ta". Those tumors which histological examination shows to have reached the lamina propria but
not gone beyond have been reserved for "T1".

     The problem of TIS as a clinical entity looms larger with each
passing year. We have not been able to characterize it nor can we
estimate its precise threat to the host. Its propensity for
extending laterally, its difficulty in visual identification, its
multifocality - these features make definition very difficult.

     A new dimension to this already heterogenous disease was
added when Melicow (6) first described it in bladders which had been

removed because of invasive carcinoma. The description was received as mildly interesting but at that time Urologists the world over were preoccupied with potentially lethal disease, the invasive carcinoma. Eisenberg et al (7) eight years later noted that it occurred with Ta and T1 lesions and when it did the results of treatment were often very poor. Nevertheless, the relatively high survival rates resulting from TUR or fulguration in patients with Ta and T1 lesions has led to no evident concern until nearly another decade had passed. By then a spate of articles concerning TIS appeared (8, 9, 10), and in them were patients with only TIS, and no other form of tumor (11). Some of these patients died of invasive carcinoma, others had cystectomy with survival, and still others had just TUR's. There is a suggestion from these reports that the more extensive the tumor at diagnosis the more likely the disease was to progress and become uncontrollable. This had not been proven, of course.

Possibly TIS was ignored because it was not always reported. Althausen et al (12) reviewed the records of 129 consecutive patients with five-year follow-ups. Twenty nine never had another tumor (Table 1). The remainder did, and thirty eight developed invasive cancer and all but eight of these died. When the slides were reviewed by Daly some of the gratuitously resected mucosa around the papillary tumor was found to be either atypical or TIS. All available blocks were recut and the results shown in Table 2. In this retrospectively analyzed group of patients, both atypia and TIS were powerful predictors for invasion.

These data argue strongly for the "field change" hypothesis. One may propose that carcinogens, not yet defined, had afflicted the urothelium creating abnormalities in cells which, upon dividing, produce neoplasms. As seen from a clinical view, this is a readily acceptable proposition. The work of Sandberg et al (13) and Falor and Ward (14) suggest that other mechanisms are functioning as well. They have studied karyotypes of superficial tumors and found that multiple tumors occurring in the same bladder may have the same marker chromosome and that recurrent tumors will also have the same markers. This suggests that at least some of the tumors we encounter are monoclonal and are arising from implants. Since selection in karyotyping may result in biased results it can only be suggested that all recurrences are due to seeding of viable cells from one initial tumor. Quite likely, a combination of events is occurring. This combination is probably influenced by therapy as well as by the biology of neoplastic diathesis.

The National Bladder Cancer Project has as its therapeutic arm Collaborative Group A. Currently ten centers are accessioning patients. A statistical center and a central pathology laboratory combine to make the Group (Table 3).

TABLE 1

Five year follow up in 129 patients with low grade,
low stage transitional cell bladder cancer

	No. Pts.	(%)
Recurrence	109	(85)
No recurrence	20	(15)
Total	129	
Non-invasion	90	(70)
Invasion	39	(30)
Total	129	

TABLE 2

Neighboring urothelium (sufficient for study in
78/129 patients)

		Invasion	
		No. of Pts.	(%)
Normal	41	3	(7)
Atypia	25	9	(36)
Carcinoma in situ	12	10	(83)
Total	78	22	

TABLE 3

National Bladder Cancer Collaborative Group A
Composition as of January 1, 1981

Chairman: George R. Prout, Jr., M.D.
Administrative Deputy: Janice Kopp, M.B.A.

Central Pathology Laboratory (CPL)*   Gilbert Friedell, M.D., Worcester, Mass.
Statistical Center (SC)**   Sidney Cutler, Ph.D., Washington, D.C.

Participating Institutions and Principal Investigators:

Johns Hopkins Hospital, Baltimore, Md. - Dr Patrick Walsh
Massachusetts General Hospital, Boston, Mass. - Dr George R. Prout, Jr.
Medical College of Virginia, Richmond, Va. - Dr Warren W. Koontz, Jr.
Roswell Park Memorial Institute, Buffalo, N.Y. - Dr Zew Wajsman
Rush-Presbyterian-St Luke's Medical Center, Chicago, Ill. - Dr Malachi Flanagan
University of California, San Diego, Calif. - Dr Joseph Schmidt
University of Iowa Hospitals & Clinics, Iowa City, Iowa - Dr Stefan Loening
University of Oregon, Portland, Ore. - Dr Harper Pearse
University of Tennessee, Memphis, Tenn. - Dr Mark Soloway
University of Wisconsin, Madison, Wis. - Dr Kenneth Cummings
Virginia Mason Clinic, Seattle, Wash. - Dr George Brannen

*   Located at St Vincents Hospital
** Located at Georgetown University

CYSTOSCOPY REPORT   **MALE**

Patient Last Name	First	Middle Initial	STAT COORD CEN USE ONLY
Institution		Patient Hospital Number	Reg. # _____ Form # _____
			Hosp. # _____ Study # _____

Date of this Cystoscopy ___/___/___ Mo Day Yr

Date of previous Cystoscopy ___/___/___ Mo Day Yr

[ ] Initial Diagnosis

Was bladder diagram from previous cystoscopy available for comparison?
[ ] -Yes   [ ] -No

[ ] Follow-up Examination   [ ] Prior Exam at Same Institution   [ ] Prior Exam at Other Institution

INSTRUCTIONS: Outline and number all tumors, suspicious areas, and selected mucosal biopsies. Report findings in table below.

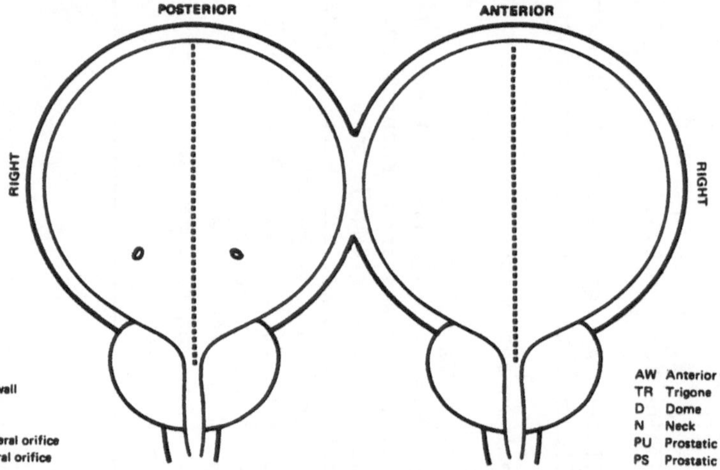

POSTERIOR   ANTERIOR

RIGHT   RIGHT

PW Posterior wall
RW Right wall
LW Left wall
RU Right ureteral orifice
LU Left ureteral orifice

AW Anterior wall
TR Trigone
D Dome
N Neck
PU Prostatic urethra
PS Prostatic substance

TUMOR OR BIOPSY SITE

NUMBER OR LETTER								
LOCATION								
PROCEDURE								
TUMOR BIOPSY								
ADJACENT TO TUMOR BIOPSY								
SUSPICIOUS AREA BIOPSY								
SELECTED MUCOSAL BIOPSY								
RESECTION								
FULGURATION								
SHAPE								
FLAT								
SESSILE								
PAPILLARY								
BULLOUS EDEMA								

Size of Largest Tumor

_____ (cm.)

BLADDER STATUS AT FOLLOW-UP

[ ] No visible tumor
[ ] Suspicious area(s)

Tumor Visible: [ ] Same site(s)
[ ] Adjacent site(s)
[ ] New site(s)
[ ] None specified

I HAVE REVIEWED THIS COMPLETED DIAGRAM AND TABLE AND CONFIRM THAT IT ACCURATELY REPRESENTS MY ENDOSCOPIC FINDINGS.

Signature _____   Date _____

Fig. 2.   Diagram of the male bladder to be completed by Urologist at cystoscopy. The diagram is laminated in plastic and supplied with a sterile pen for use in the Operating Room.

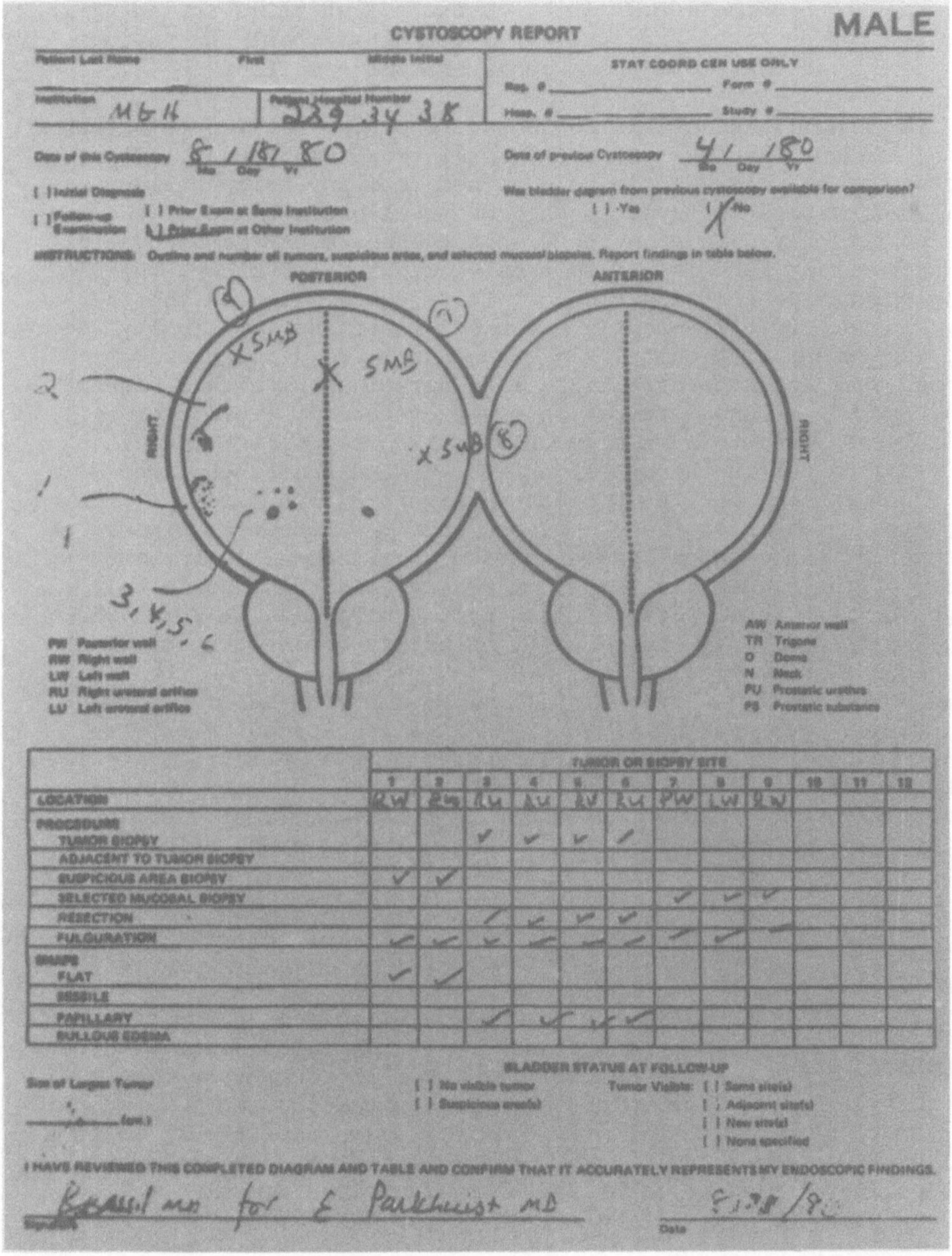

Fig. 3. Photograph of a completed cystoscopy report.

It is the first two protocols that are relevant here (3, 15).
They have been consolidated into Protocol 1A which is now in use.
Briefly, the protocol provides for the evaluation of the patient,
the tumor, and the field from whence the tumor arises.

We found it acceptable to compare the results of cytology from
saline bladder washings and urine obtained at cystoscopy. We also
agreed that biopsies should be obtained from any tumor present as
well as from those lateral to each ureteral orifice and in the mid-
line posteriorly. We soon found that the shape of the bladder did
not necessarily lend itself to precise mapping. Further, the
Pathologist's description did not always correlate with the operator's note. Put differently, we had investigator difficulty and
data management difficulty. To correct this we developed a
diagram that could be sterilized in a packet along with a sterile
pen (Fig. 2). These were put on every cystoscopy table when a
patient was found to have a tumor. We then stipulated that it had
to be filled out in the operating room. Note that there are
descriptive sites for ten biopsies. Figure 3 is an example of a
completed sheet. Next we stipulated that the Pathologist named as
a member of the clinical research team was responsible for the
review of the slides and pathology reports and they should be
congruent with the operative note and the diagram. We found that
this was the only way that data might arrive at the CPL and SC and
not require interpretation.

We also learned that saline washings produce superior pre-
parations (15). Nevertheless, in analyzing the patient it is wise
to be ever alert to discordant results. If the urinary cytology
is positive and the saline cytology is negative, careful evaluation of the upper tracts is in order including catheterization of
both ureters to obtain cytological specimens as well as pyelograms.

It should be remembered that well differentiated tumors do
not produce a high yield of positive cytology. Therefore, when the
tumor biopsy is positive for a grade 1 lesion and the cytology is
positive, it is necessary for the Urologist to review the cytological findings. If fronds of well differentiated cells are found
and the cytology is read as positive, then little further is
necessary. On the other hand, the cytological specimens may con-
tain anaplastic cells while the only positive tumor biopsy is of a
well differentiated tumor. This suggests that TIS is present in
that patient's bladder. The papillary tumor was visible, the
TIS was not.

Finally, it should be emphasized that this longitudinal program
is an hypothesis-generating one. We can identify some obvious
studies, e.g., saline bladder washings versus urine for cytology,
different doses of thio-TEPA, systematic evaluation of cytotoxic

drugs, but one of the major goals is to study and classify bladder carcinoma as it has never been before. Some of the results of the protocols we have followed appear elsewhere in this publication.

REFERENCES

1. G.R. Prout Jr., Introduction: Management (control) of early bladder lesions, Cancer Res. 37: 2891-2893 (1977).
2. National Bladder Cancer Collaborative Group A, Development of a strategy for a longitudinal study of patients with bladder cancer, Cancer Res. 37: 2898-2907 (1977).
3. National Bladder Cancer Collaborative Group A, Surveillance, initial assessment and subsequent progress of patients with superficial bladder cancer in a prospective longitudinal study, Cancer Res. 37: 2907-2911 (1977).
4. H.J. Jewett and G.H. Strong, Infiltrating carcinoma of the bladder: relation of depth of penetration of the bladder wall to incidence of local extension and metastases, J. Urol. 55: 366-372 (1946).
5. V.F. Marshall, The relation of the preoperative estimate to the pathologic demonstration of the extent of vesical neoplasms, J. Urol. 68: 714-723 (1952).
6. M.M. Melicow, Histological study of vesical urothelium intervening between gross neoplasms in total cystectomy, J. Urol. 68: 261-265 (1952).
7. R.B. Eisenberg, R.B. Roth and M.H. Schweinsberg, Bladder tumors and associated proliferative mucosal lesions, J. Urol. 84: 544-549 (1960).
8. D.C. Utz, K.A. Hanash and G.M. Farrow, The plight of the patient with carcinoma-in-situ of the bladder, J. Urol. 103: 160-168 (1970).
9. R.O.K. Schade and J. Swinney, Pre-cancerous changes in bladder epithelium, Lancet 2: 943-950 (1968).
10. M.R. Melamed, H. Grabstald and W.F. Whitmore Jr., Carcinoma-in-situ of the bladder: clinico-pathologic study of a case with suggested approach to detection, J. Urol. 96: 466-469 (1966).
11. D.C. Utz and H. Zincke, The masquerade of bladder carcinoma-in-situ as interstitial cystitis, Trans. Amer. Assoc. Genitourinary Surg. 65: 64-69 (1973).
12. A.F. Althausen, G.R. Prout Jr., and J.J. Daly, Non-invasive papillary carcinoma of the bladder associated with carcinoma in situ, J. Urol. 116: 575-580 (1976).
13. A.A. Sandberg, Chromosome markers and progression in bladder cancer, Cancer Res. 37: 2950-2956 (1977).
14. W.H. Falor and R.M. Ward, Prognosis in well differentiated non-invasive carcinoma of the bladder based on chromosomal analysis, Surg. Gynec. Obstet. 144: 515-521 (1977).
15. National Bladder Cancer Collaborative Group A, Cytology and histopathology of bladder cancer cases in a prospective longitudinal study, Cancer Res. 37: 2911-2915 (1977).

BLADDER CANCER - SURGERY

W. VAHLENSIECK

University Hospital
Bonn
GERMANY

SUMMARY

The choice of surgical approach in the management of bladder
cancer depends on the localisation, number, TNM-stage, histology and
grade of malignancy of the tumors.   The indications and possibilities
of transurethral resection, laser and cryotherapy treatment will be
discussed.   At the moment TUR is the most common treatment for T1-2,
No, Mo tumors but should always be carried out in association with
mapping (multiple cold biopsies).   The incidence of recurrences can
probably be reduced by adjuvant intravesical cytotoxic therapy,
especially in cases with multiple tumors, if cystectomy is not
indicated or is not possible.

The indications and methods of open operative treatment are discussed.   In all cases a pelvic lymphadenectomy should first be done
for the purpose of staging.   If a T3-4, No, Mo stage is confirmed,
transvesical electroresection, partial bladder resection or cystectomy
may be sufficient to cure the patient.   If there is nodal involvement (category N+) lymphadenectomy and cystectomy leads to a reduction
of tumor mass and prevents pain, but has to be followed by adjuvant
treatment.

INTRODUCTION

The operative treatment of urinary bladder tumors is essentially
influenced by localisation, number, TNM stage, histology and grade of
malignancy.

In Table 1 established treatment modalities as well as those
methods under investigation are summarised.   As far as any operative

TABLE 1

BLADDER CANCER - POSSIBLE SURGICAL APPROACH

I.   Transurethral treatment

      1.   TUR
      2.   Laser therapy
      3.   Cryosurgery

II. Open operative treatment

      1.   Transvesical resection
      2.   Segmental resection
      3.   Cystectomy

treatment is possible, the best procedure has to be determined on
the basis of the results of careful diagnostic evaluation.

TRANSURETHRAL TREATMENT

Transurethral Resection (TUR)

Without consideration of histology and grade of malignancy, TUR
is the method of choice in category T1 tumors, e.g. tumors which are
confined to the mucosa without infiltration of the muscularis.

The percentage of T1 tumors certainly varies in different
hospitals due to the selection of patients.   Evaluating our 231
bladder cancer cases from 1963-72, we found 101 T1 No Mo tumours (44%)
(Table 2).   The evaluation of the T1 category is achieved by the
technique of resection.   After resection of the exophytic portion
of the tumor, the tumor base is deeply resected.   If the pathologist
does not find any tumor cells in the deeply resected material, a T1
category has to be assumed.   Altwein et al (4) reported a 56% five-
year survival for T1 tumors whereas that in the series of Mauermayer
and Tauber was 42% (16).

Of the 101 T1 No Mo patients we found a five-year survival of
68% after TUR.   Analysing the differing and unsatisfactory results,
attention should first of all be directed to the grade of malignancy.
According to Altwein et al (4) and Barnes et al (5) a five-year
survival rate of 66 and 81% respectively can be expected in well
differentiated T1 tumors, whereas with the moderately differentiated
and anaplastic lesions the rates fall to 59 and 30% respectively
(Table 3).   The question is how can we obtain better results?

A very important role is played by mapping, in which serial
multiple-site biopsies are performed at the time of TUR.   Soloway

TABLE 2

PERCENTAGE OF DIFFERENT STAGES IN 231 BLADDER TUMORS

Stage	n	%
T1 NO MO	101	43.7
T2 Nx MO	28	12.1
T3 Nx MO	38	16.5
T4 Nx MO	26	11.3
T4 N1-4 MO	18	7.8
T4 N1-4 M1a-d	20	8.6
	231	100 %

TABLE 3

SURVIVAL RATES IN RELATION TO STAGE

Stage	n	Survival (Years)				
		1	2	3	4	5+
T1, NO, MO	101	91/97 (94%)	76/89 (85%)	60/75 (80%)	53/72 (74%)	46/48 (68%)
T2, NX, MO	28	22/24 (91%)	16/23 (70%)	10/20 (50%)	8/18 (44%)	5/17 (30%)
T3, NX, MO	38	19/37 (51%)	15/35 (43%)	10/28 (36%)	4/20 (20%)	2/15 (13%)
T4, NX, MO	26	10/25 (40%)	5/25 (20%)	1/23 (4%)	1/17 (6%)	1/10 (10%)
T4, N1-4, MO	18	6/14 (43%)	3/12 (25%)	2/11 (18%)	-	-
T4, N1-4, M1 a-d	20	5/12 (41%)	1/9 (11%)	-	-	-

et al (21) showed that approximately 10% of patients with bladder
tumors had carcinomas in the apparently normal portion of the bladder
at the time of tumor resection; another 20% had epithelial anomalies.
Althausen et al (2) have already shown that in cases with epithelial
alterations an increasing incidence of invasive cancer may be expected
during the course of the disease.   On control biopsies every three
months over one year, Soloway et al (21) showed an increasing rate of
occult carcinoma (30%) and of epithelial atypias (50%).

These facts stress the necessity of mapping of the bladder mucosa
at the primary tumor resection.   In patients with multiple occult
carcinomas TUR alone cannot be justified.   In G1 tumors we would
favour local cytostatic chemotherapy; in G2 and G3 tumors cystectomy
seems to be necessary.   Furthermore, prognosis can definitely be
improved by early recognition and optimal treatment of recurrences,
which according to Altwein et al (4), occur in G1 tumors in 22.7%
and in G2-3 tumors in 57.7% of the cases.   Also important is the
observation of Gilbert et al (14) that recurrences exhibit a greater
anaplasia than the primary tumor in one quarter of the cases.

Because of this, the question of adjunctive local cytostatic
chemotherapy deserves special attention in the hope that the prognosis
may be improved.   Certainly Catalona (7) correctly emphasized the
point that many questions are still unsolved.   We have only scanty
experience with adriamycin and mitomycin C and, by local application
of thiotepa employing 60 mg. for 4-8 weeks either in water solution
or in a long adhering emulsion, we were unable to achieve a definite
improvement of the recurrence rate.

On the other hand, after nonspecific stimulation of the cellular
immune response by BCG subsequent to radical TUR, we have so far
observed a very low recurrence rate (Table 4).   However, one has to
await the results of treatment of a larger group of patients before
drawing definite conclusions.

Independent of the question of the effectiveness of local cytostatic chemotherapy, regular supervision is essential for the early
recognition of recurrences.   For that purpose, starting three months
after TUR, urinary cytology should be performed every 6-8 weeks.
The method is specific and devoid of stress for the patient, and the
expenditure seems worthwhile, especially as tumor recurrences cannot
be excluded if one looks only for red cells in the urine either microscopically or by test papers (sangurtest).

One problem is that urinary cytologyis not generally available
as a routine method.   If cytology is not available the urine should
be examined for red cells at least every four weeks or the paper test
should be done 1-3 times per week during the first year after TUR.
If a test is positive, an immediate cystourethroscopy is indicated;
otherwise it should be performed every three months.   All suspicious

TABLE 4

RESULTS OF CHEMOIMMUNE PROPHYLAXIS IN 25 PATIENTS
WITH Tl GI-III TUMORS

(from H.-D. Adolphs and J. Thiele: presented at the
4th Congress of Eur. Urol. Ass., Athens, 1980)

No. of Patients	Recurrence	Postoperative time (months)				
		0-6	7-12	13-18	19-24	24
25	no	9	6	3	3	3
	yes	1				

areas of the mucosa should be resected and mapping should also be
included.   During the second year after TUR, the urine should be
tested at least once a month and cystourethroscopy must be performed
every six months.   If no recurrence is noted during the first two
years, cystourethroscopy once per year is sufficient.

Barnes et al (5) showed that the five year survival rate in T2
tumors after TUR alone is 75% for highly differentiated tumors and
21% for anaplastic lesions.   In addition to the known tendency to
recurrences this bad prognosis might be the result of micrometastases
already established in regional lymph nodes, as shown by Prout (18).
Therefore, in T2 No Mo tumors of category Gl, systemic cytostatic
treatment or external radiotherapy should be considered.   In cases
with G2 and G3 tumors cystectomy alone might improve the prognosis.

In T3 and T4 tumors, TUR is considered as a palliative treatment
for reduction of tumor bulk in connection with radio- or cytostatic
therapy, if other forms of treatment are not indicated.

Laser Treatment

This is still in the experimental stage and we do not have any
experience with this technique.   Lasers are light sources.   The
emitted light exhibits parallelism, high monochromasia, complete
coherence, and high energy density.   For the transurethral treatment
of bladder tumors, CO_2, argon-, and neodym-YAG (an yttrium-aluminium-
garnet crystal) lasers have been tested.   Hofstetter et al (15)
reported a penetration and coagulation by the laser beam of 3-4 mm.
using the neodym-YAG model with 45 watt.   This means that with a
laser of this efficiency only Tl and T2 tumors can be destroyed.
An increase of power beyond 45 watt is, however, possible resulting
in transmural necrosis, suitable for the destruction of T3 tumors.
In this situation, however, there is the danger of injuring the
adjacent bowel.   This complication can only be avoided if

simultaneous laparoscopy is performed to ensure protection of the
bowel.   Hofstetter et al (15) consider the neodym-YAG laser
advantageous in that without anesthesia (but perhaps with sedation)
T1-T2 tumors can quickly be destroyed without blood loss and without
postoperative catheterization.   On the other hand this very sensitive equipment is expensive.   In addition, TUR does not put much
more stress on the patient.   Furthermore, fractionated TUR allows
determination of the tumor stage.   Another disadvantage of laser
treatment is the necessity to resect exophytic tumors larger than
2 cm. in diameter by TUR, before treating the tumor bed by laser.

Cryotherapy

Since there are no reports on the results of treatment of large
numbers of patients it would appear that cryotherapy does not have
any advantage over the established treatment modalities.   Therefore,
I do not want to go into further details of this treatment, which,
of course, does not deny the fact that this technique occasionally
may help to alleviate heavy bleeding.

OPEN OPERATIVE TREATMENT

Transvesical Resection

Transvesical tumor resection with special loops has occasionally
been used for resection of large multicentric exophytic tumors.   We
followed 20 patients treated in this way and found that two-thirds
of the patients derived benefit for one or two years;   ultimately
only three out of 15 (20%) survived five years.   The technique is
only useful as a palliative treatment and should only be considered
for reduction of tumor bulk with subsequent radiotherapy, to increase
bladder capacity, or for the treatment of intermittent haematuria if
partial resection or cystectomy is excluded for any reason.

Segmental Resection

Partial resection is also controversial although this technique
has definite advantages in so far as urinary diversion is not
required.

In our 27 cases (Table 5) we found that approximately two-thirds
of the patients (17/26) survived the first year.   However, from the
second year the rate dropped and one third were alive after five
years (5/15).   Faysal and Freiha (13) reported a recurrence rate of
78%.   The rates of recurrences and survival in stage A tumors in
relation to the tumor grade (20,25) are also very interesting whilst
the poor survival in the more advanced cases is also clear from the
other figures in Table 5.   In these circumstances the indications
for partial resection are probably limited.   An improvement of
prognosis can only be expected if:

    (a)   Preliminary evaluation and pelvic lymph node dissection exclude both regional and distant metastases.

    (b)   Partial resection is really radical.   This means that the resection has to be at least 3-4 cm. away from the tumor and that the margin must be tumor free on histological frozen section.

TABLE 5

BLADDER CANCER - RESULTS OF SEGMENTAL RESECTION

Author		Recurrence	5-Year Survival
Cummings et al. 1978 (n = 101)	Stage 0, A, B1		83%
		49%	
	B2, C		27%
Schoborg et al. 1979 (n = 45)	Stage A GI/II	28%	86%
	Stage A GIII/IV	100%	40%
Altwein et al. 1980 (n = 50)	Stage 0, A, B1		56%
		62%	
	Stage B2, C, D		23%
Vahlensieck (n = 27)	Stage B2, C	-	33%

Better results may be obtained as stated by Schoborg et al (20) if one does not hesitate to perform a subtotal cystectomy with re-implantation of the ureter (Fig. 1).   To cover the defect, one can use lyophilized dura or one may wait for regeneration to occur.   In all our cases (n = 19) treated by subtotal resection and subsequent regeneration, we have observed both normal micturition and a normal bladder capacity.   An outstanding example of this technique is one of our patients who, 12 years after subtotal bladder resection with partial resection and re-implantation of the ureter and open regener-ation, survives tumor free with normal micturition.

Cystectomy

The indications for cystectomy are clear, and include multiple primary tumors, tumors which infiltrate the bladder wall and invasive recurrences.   The varying reports on the five-year survival seem to be contradictory.   The figures range from 53 - 83% for patients with superficial muscle invasion and from 0 - 57% for those with deep infiltration (1).   Prospective studies should clarify the situation as to the influence of stage, grade of malignancy, age, general condition of the patient and the mode of urinary diversion.   There is no doubt in our minds however, that the absence of metastases should be proved by lymphadenectomy before cystectomy is undertaken.

The question of whether preoperative radiotherapy leads to better results than cystectomy alone is still open.   Whereas Van der Werf-Messing (22), Whitmore et al (24), Chan and Johnson (8) reported excellent results with preoperative radiotherapy, Blackard and Byar (6), Prout (17), Daughtry et al (12), Clark (9) and Vinnicombe and Abercrombie (23) did not notice that preoperative radiation conferred any advantage compared with the course of the disease after cystectomy alone.   Recent observations on downstaging and the type of tumor which responds to irradiation seem to indicate a possible solution to this problem.   Prout et al (19) found no evidence of tumor in the cystectomy specimen in many patients after radiotherapy with 4000-4500 rad.   They were also able to demonstrate that nodular tumors regressed much better than the papillary forms.   Crawford and Skinner (10)investigating cystectomy specimens after a full course of radio-therapy (salvage cystectomy) showed that patients with radiosensitive tumors either had no bladder tumor or only superficial tumors (i.e. downstaged) with a five-year survival rate of 63%.   On the other hand in patients with persisting (radioresistant) invasive tumors, a five-year survival of only 19% could be achieved.   One has to agree with Catalona (7) that in the 55 - 65% of patients whose tumors persist due to radioresistance, radiation might be disadvantageous since it could facilitate the development of metastases as a result of both an impairment in the patient's general condition and an increase of time for dissemination whereas immediate cystectomy without radiation might be curative.   Thus, for the moment, we perform cystectomy alone

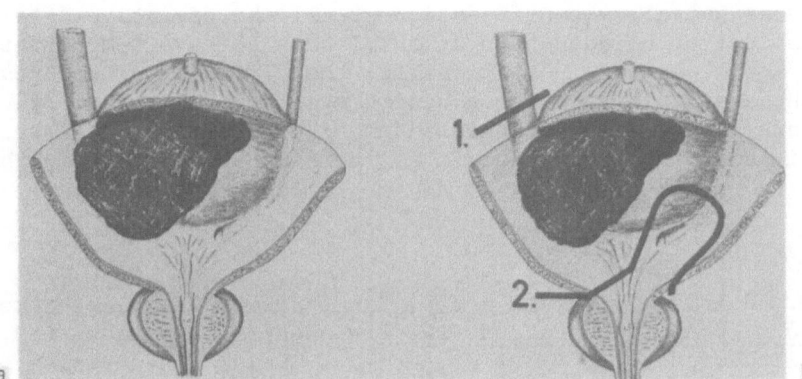

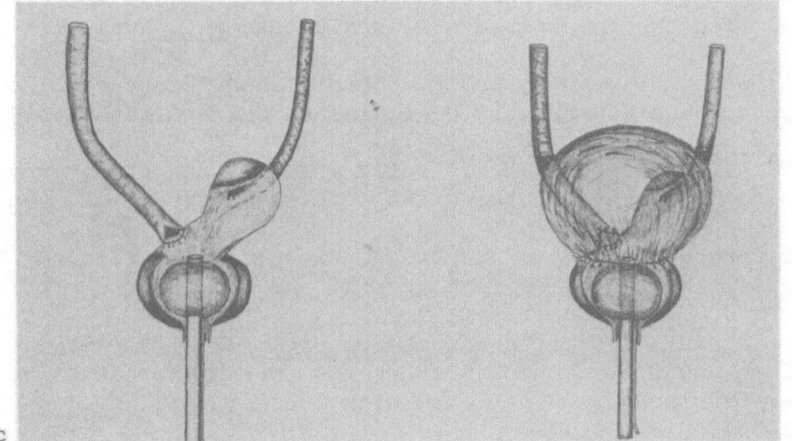

Fig. 1. a.   Large bladder tumor extending to the right ureteric
             orifice.
        b.   1. Subtotal bladder resection with removal of the right
             ureteric orifice and partial resection of the right
             distal ureter; 2. Residual portion of bladder; in males
             prostatectomy is also carried out.
        c.   Reimplantation of the right ureter, if possible with
             antireflux mechanism.
        d.   The defect is covered with lyophilized dura or
             spontaneous regeneration is awaited.

in patients with G1 and G2 tumors whereas in G3 tumors cystectomy is preceded by irradiation.

Time does not allow consideration of all the operative details in the treatment of bladder tumors, but I hope to have demonstrated that there are clear-cut indications for the different procedures and that the available techniques become ever more satisfactory. By this means and by using planned adjunctive treatment modalities in appropriate cases, the prognosis may perhaps be improved in the future.

REFERENCES

1. H. -D. Adolphs, J. Thiele and W. Vahlensieck, Harnblasentumoren, Fortschr. Urol. Nephrol. Bd. 12, Steinkopff, Darmstadt, (1979).
2. A.F. Althausen, G.R. Prout Jr. and J.J. Daly, Non-invasive Papillary Carcinoma of the Bladder Associated with Carcinoma In Situ, J. Urol. 116: 575 (1976).
3. J.E. Altwein, T. Klotz and G.H. Jacobi, Stellenwert der Blasenteilresektion zur Therapie des Blasentumors, Akt. Urol. 11: 351 (1980).
4. J.E. Altwein, K.E. Kurth and R. Hohenfellner, Blasencarcinom: Therapeutisches Konzept der Urologischen Universitätsklinik Mainz, Urologe A, 16: 180 (1977).
5. R.E. Barnes, A.L. Dick, H.L. Hadley and O.L. Johnston, Survival Following Transurethral Resection of Bladder Carcinoma, Cancer Res. 37: 2895 (1977).
6. C.E. Blackard, D.B. Byar and VACURG, Results of a Clinical Trial of Surgery and Radiation in Stages II and III Carcinoma of the Bladder, J. Urol. 108: 875 (1972).
7. W.J. Catalona, Bladder Carcinoma, J. Urol. 123: 35 (1980).
8. R.C. Chan and D.E. Johnson, Integrated Therapy for Invasive Bladder Carcinoma. Experience with 108 Patients, Urology 12: 549 (1978).
9. P.B. Clark, Radical Cystectomy for Carcinoma of the Bladder, Brit. J. Urol. 50: 492 (1978).
10. E.D. Crawford and D.G. Skinner, Salvage Cystectomy After Irradiation Failure, J. Urol. 123: 32 (1980).
11. K.B. Cummings, J.T. Mason, R.J. Correa Jr. and R.P. Gibbons, Segmental Resection in the Management of Bladder Carcinoma, J. Urol. 119: 56 (1978).
12. J.D. Daughtry, L.P. Susan, B.H. Stewart and R.S. Straffon, Ileal Conduit and Cystectomy: a 10 Year Retrospective Study of Ileal Conduits Performed in Conjunction with Cystectomy and with a Minimum 5 Year Follow Up, J. Urol. 118: 556 (1977).
13. M.H. Faysal and F.S. Freiha, Evaluation of Partial Cystectomy for Carcinoma of Bladder, Urology 14: 352 (1979).

14. H.A. Gilbert, J.L. Logan, A.R. Kagan, H.A. Friedman, J.K. Cove,
     M. Fox, T.M. Muldoon, Y.W. Lonni, J.H. Rowe, J.F. Cooper,
     H. Nussbaum, P. Chan, A. Rao and A. Starr, The Natural History
     of Papillary Transitional Cell Carcinoma of the Bladder and its
     Treatment in an Unselected Population on the Basis of Histology
     Grading, J. Urol. 119: 488 (1978).
15. A. Hofstetter, E. Schmiedt and G. Staehler, Stellungnahme zur
     Arbeit von E. Matouschek, Urologe B 20: 25 (1980).
16. W. Mauermayer and R. Tauber, Die Tumoren der Harnblase - Indik-
     ation, Technik und Ergebnisse der Transurethralen Therapie,
     Urologe A 16: 185 (1977).
17. G.R. Prout Jr., The Surgical Management of Bladder Carcinoma,
     Urol. Clin. N. Amer. 3: 149 (1976).
18. G.R. Prout Jr., The Role of Surgery in the Potentially Curative
     Treatment of Bladder Carcinoma, Cancer Res. 37: 2764 (1977).
19. G.R. Prout Jr., P.P. Griffin and W.U. Shipley, Bladder Carcinoma
     as a Systemic Disease, Cancer 43: 2532 (1979).
20. T.W. Schoborg, J.L. Sapolsky and C.W. Lewis Jr., Carcinoma of
     Bladder Treated by Segmental Resection, J. Urol. 122: 473 (1979).
21. M.S. Soloway, W. Murphy, M.K. Rao and C. Cox, Serial Multiple-
     Site Biopsies in Patients with Bladder Cancer, J. Urol. 120: 57
     (1978).
22. B. Van der Werf-Messing, Proceedings: Carcinoma of the Bladder
     Treated by Preoperative Irradiation Followed by Cystectomy,
     Cancer 32: 1084 (1973).
23. J. Vinnicombe and G.F. Abercrombie, Total Cystectomy - A Review,
     Brit. J. Urol. 50: 488 (1978).
24. W.F. Whitmore Jr., M.A. Batata, M.A. Ghoneim, H. Grabstald and
     A. Unal, Radical Cystectomy With or Without Prior Irradiation
     in the Treatment of Bladder Cancer, J. Urol. 118: 184 (1977).
25. J.L. Williams, J.C. Hammonds and N. Saunders, T1 Bladder Tumors,
     Brit. J. Urol. 49: 663 (1977).

RADIATION THERAPY OF CARCINOMA OF THE URINARY BLADDER

B VAN DER WERF-MESSING

Rotterdamsch Radio-Therapeutisch Instituut
Rotterdam
The Netherlands

Radiation therapy has a significant place in the treatment of carcinoma of the urinary bladder, not only as a palliative tool in cases with metastases, where pain can be relieved and dangerous sequelae such as fractures and paralysis can be prevented, but also as curative treatment.

Curative radiotherapy is mainly indicated in infiltrating bladder malignancies, i.e. category T1-, T2-, T3- and T4- carcinomas, without distant metastases - category MO according to the international classification of the UICC (1)

As bladder cancers are usually not very radiosensitive but commonly remain localised for a relatively long period, interstitial radium implant given with curative intent is the treatment of choice in the Rotterdam Radio-Therapy Institute (R.R.T.I.). By this approach a very high dose can be given to the growth and adjacent tissues without are unacceptable radiation dose to the patient's adjacent healthy organs. The indications for radium implantation are a bladder cancer of category T1,T2 and T3 without evidence of distant metastases. The diameter of the growth should not exceed 5 cms in order to avoid unacceptable necrosis and the general condition of the patient has to be compatible with supra-pubic intervention as the radium needles are inserted by this route. After implantation of the needles the bladder is closed immediately; a three dimensional reconstruction of each implant is made in order to calculate the appropriate application time, i.e. the time in which a tumour killing dose will be delivered. After this time the needles are removed by pulling the threads to which they are attached; no anaesthesia is required for this procedure.

As the radium implant is done through the open bladder, the opportunity is given to compare the surgical T-category with the clinical staging. It turns out that in the T1-category the surgical T-category corresponds to the clinical one in more than 80%. The clinical T2-category is correct in 80%, the main mistake being understaging. However, according to international rules, all T2-growths remain in the T2-category for further assessment. In the T3-category the staging is most correct - 90%.

After radium implant actuarial uncorrected survival rates after five years are 75% in 164 cases of the T1-category, 55% in 313 cases of the T2-category and 25% in 129 cases of the T3-category.

The complication rate in 606 patients treated with a radium implant is about 9%, 2% being lethal mainly due to pulmonary embolism after operation (nine cases) and due to urosepsis during follow-up (two cases). Alive with complications are 7%. Of these 11 cases had to undergo subsequent urinary diversion in order to overcome the complications.

As at the beginning scar-implants were noted during the follow-up, it was decided to add 3 x 350 rad to the scar after healing of the wound. Ten years later this post-radium scar irradiation was substituted by preoperative irradiation, 3 x 350 rad being given to the true pelvis. By doing so it was hoped to prevent scar implants and at the same time to reduce the incidence of iatrogenic metastases. It turned out that in the T1-category no scar-implants were seen at all, hence any additional external irradiation in this T-category was abandoned. In the T2-category scar-implant incidence decreased from 6% without external irradiation to zero after preoperative irradiation. In the T3-category the incidence of scar-implants also decreased, from 23% without external irradiation to zero after preoperative irradiation.

Not only were scar-implants influenced by preoperative irradiation, but also the incidence of distant metastases. In the T1-category again no influence of external irradiation could be demonstrated, the incidence of metastases being about 10%. In the T2-category the incidence of distant metastases decreased from 25% without additional external irradiation to 10% after preoperative irradiation. The corresponding incidence of metastases in the T3-category was 45% and 10%.

The effect of this preoperative irradiation (3 x 350 rad to the true pelvis) had a significant bearing on prognosis in the T3-category. If no additional external irradiation was given the uncorrected five year survival rate was about 10% whereas after 3 x 350 rad preoperative irradiation it rose to 35%.

During a period of about five years, prior to the radium implant and when the bladder was already opened, a biopsy was taken from the healthy mucosa at about 2 cms distance from the clinically evident growth. Carcinoma was found in 17% of the T1-category, in about 13% of the T2-category and in 34% of the T3-category. However, this finding had no bearing on the incidence of local recurrence. In the T1 category the local recurrence rate was about 18% in all groups disregarding the biopsy findings at 2 cms; in the T2-category the same finding applied, 15% recurred locally, again disregarding the findings at biopsy; in the T3-category the same situation - about 34% local recurrence rate. Hence it can be speculated that the radium implant might also have an impact on a patient's tumour containing bladder tissue, adjacent to and collapsing onto the implanted area.

If patients were not suitable for a radium implant a full course of external irradiation was aimed at. By this method a dose which is biologically much lower than the dose given by radium implant was delivered to the malignancy. Also more healthy tissues and organs were exposed to this irradiation. Usually, at the R.R.T.I. irradiátion was given by three fields. A total dose of 6500 to 7000 rad was delivered by daily fractions of 200 rad.

Actuarial uncorrected survival rates are disappointing. After three years nobody who presented with distant metastases at the time of treatment was alive. Patients with T1- and T2- growths had about 25% chance of being cured after three years. This cure rate dropped to 20% and 15% in the T3- and T4- category respectively. After five years cure rates are more or less comparable. However, this group of 1102 patients treated by external irradiation also contained many patients who were in too poor a condition to receive a full course of irradiation or even to be staged appropriately. Those who could be treated to the full dose had a roughly 10% better prognosis in each T-category.

Of 978 patients who received a full course of irradiation, 27 developed complications (2.8%). Of these, 17 were lethal (1.7%). The most common complications were contracted bladder, chronic cystitis and rectal bleeding. However, the incidence of complications has decreased with improved technique. On the other hand, if more patients had lived a longer time the observable incidence might have been higher (2).

As the results of a full course of external irradiation were not satisfactory it was decided to replace a full course of external irradiation by preoperative irradiation followed by cystectomy in those patients who could tolerate it. The indications for this type of treatment were bladder cancer category T1, T2, T3 without evidence of distant metastases. Of course the general condition of the patient had to permit surgery. It was decided to give a dose of

4000 rad to the true pelvis in a period of four weeks by daily
fractions of 200 rad. The treatment was followed by simple cystectomy, i.e. no lymph node desection, as soon as possible.

The actuarial uncorrected survival rate up to ten years was
about 40% in all T-categories. As treatment mortality was still
considerable (about 6%) it was decided to apply this treatment
modality mainly to patients with category T3 tumours. The further
analysis of the data is focussed on this T-category.

When the cystectomy specimen was examined it turned out that in
68% of 141 cases the T-category had been reduced to a lower T-category
(T3 → P0, Pis, P1, P2); this reduction of depth of infiltration is
attributed to the preoperative irradiation and apparently it also
contributes to a better survival. In 43 cases in which T-category
reduction did not occur the ten year survival was about 25%. When
the growth had been reduced from T3 to a P2 (30 cases) survival
after five years was about 50% and after ten years 35%. In 66 cases
of reduction of the T3 growth to Po, Pis or P1, five year uncorrected
survival was more than 70%, and after ten years about 60%.

This improvement of survival could be attributed to the influence of the external irradiation on the lymph nodes as these are not
removed whilst the primary is automatically removed by cystectomy.
Of patients with no evidence of T-reduction 40% died subsequently
with clinical evidence of lymph node involvement whereas this applied
only to 7% of the patients with T-reduction. Also the incidence of
other metastases, without evidence of lymph node involvement, was
higher (90%) in the group which remained P3 as compared with the
group where T-reduction was observed (7%).

The various tumour and host factors which influenced the
prognosis adversely were (i) increasing age, (ii) a low degree of
differentiation mainly because of the increased risk of distant
metastases being present at the time of initial treatment, (iii)
a pathological IVP also slightly increased the risk, as did (iv)
a large preoperative irradiation filed, mainly in the older age
group. (v) Delay of cystectomy also had a bad influence on survival,
probably because delay implied a non-optimal condition of the
patient. (vi) The most important adverse prognostic factor was an
absence of T-reduction, as evident in the cystectomy specimen. For
this reason patients without proven T-reduction and who are in a
relatively good condition now receive elective Cis-platinum therapy
after the operation.

As the T-reduction is apparently of the utmost importance, we
attempted to assess T-reduction prior to cystectomy, after finishing
the external irradiation. After 4000 rad a T3-growth could still
be felt clinically in 64 cases. This turned out to be correct in
41%; but in the remainder, although a mass was still felt by

bimanual palpation, this turned out to be fibrosis in the cystectomy
specimen. Where the T-category after 4000 rad appeared to be reduced
to T1 or T2 (32 cases) this turned out to be correct in 94% of cases
and only twice was there still a P3-growth in the cystectomy specimen.
Hence, if T-reduction is felt, cystectomy can be proposed with confidence as the prognosis will be good. If T-reduction is not felt,
uncertainty about the prognosis remains. If may be that assessment
of acute phase reactant proteins, a study being done now, will contribute to predicting T-reduction prior to cystectomy (4).

If the results of the various types of curative treatment are
compared, it has to be realised that the indications, as far as
tumour and host conditions are concerned, vary in the different
groups. However, it is evident that the radium implant gives the
best prognosis in the T1-category. Hence, wherever possible a
radium implant should be undertaken. In the T2-category the same
applies. If the patient with the T3-growth is not suitable for a
radium implant he probably should undergo cystectomy instead of
external irradiation if he can tolerate that procedure, since in
the T3-category those who underwent cystectomy had the best prognosis.

In an attempt to improve prognosis in the T3-category a new
radium implant technique has been introduced at the R.R.T.I. for
growths not exceeding a diameter of 5 cms. External irradiation as
in the case of cystectomy was combined with a radium implant at
a reduced dose, hoping, by doing so, to combine the beneficial
influence of 4000 rad external irradiation on the lymph nodes with
conservation of the bladder. A three year uncorrected actuarial
survival rate of 65% in 28 cases with a T3-growth justifies contin-
uation of this approach (5).

About ten years ago some urologists limited treatment of T1-
growths to transurethral resection (TUR) only, if they were convinced
that the whole growth had been removed. In case of doubt, and
usually in patients with poorly differentiated growths, an additional
radium implant was given. Those urologists who were convinced that
radium implant was the best treatment did not always remove the
growth completely but limited it to a biopsy and to removal of the
exophytic part (the requirement for assessing the T-category according to the UICC). Data about the follow up were collected prospectively. Hence, though the following analysis does not represent a
prospective trial, any bias in the selection of cases is towards
"worse cases" in the Radium-group. The analysis includes only
patients with localised T1-growths and a small group of patients
with two or three T1-growths in one area which could be implanted
or have been implanted by radium.

The intercurrent death-corrected actuarial survival of 195
patients treated with radium is about 75% after five years and, for
144 patients of the TUR-group, is about 70%. After ten years the

percentage for the Radium-group is 70% and for the TUR-group is
about 35%. This is a statistically significant difference (P =
0.0002).

The five year relapse-free period for the Radium-group is 80%,
whereas it is only about 20% for the TUR-group. The same differences
are noted if the cases are subdivided according to the histological
degree of differentiation. In the Radium-group those with a high
degree of differentiation had a bladder relapse free period of 60
months in 90%; this decreased to 85% in patients with poorly differentiated lesions. In the TUR-group the relapse-free period at five
years for the same groups is only about 30% and 10% respectively.
The structure of the growth had no bearing on the relapse-free
period after radium implant, whereas after TUR only papillary
growths had about a 25% chance of remaining relapse-free up to five
years; for solid browths this chance was only about 10%. In 75% of
the TUR-group at least one recurrence was noted. This first recurrence was in a higher T-category than the original tumour in 22% of
the cases. In the Radium-group only 18% had a recurrence and only
1.5% of first recurrences had a higher T-category.

In the TUR-group 51% had to undergo up to three subsequent
TURs; in the Radium-group only 14.5%. Patients treated with TUR only
required 4 - 7 subsequent TURs in 21%, whereas this applied only to
2.5% of those treated with radium. Seven to more than 10 subsequent
TURs were done in 5% of the TUR-group and in none of the Radium-group.

In the Radium-group nearly 100% remained free of multiple recurrences during a follow-up period of five years, whereas in the
TUR-group only about 60% did so. Because of uncontrollable multiple
recurrences or because of recurrence in a higher T-category, about
60% of the TUR-group had to undergo severe treatment within ten
years, severe treatment being a full course of external irradiation
or cystectomy. In the Radium-group this was necessary in 20% of
patients only.

During follow-up metastases developed in 20% of the Radium-
group and in 50% of those treated by TUR, mainly after recurrence
in a higher T-category (3). In view of these results the majority
of Rotterdam urologists now consider TUR as the only treatment for
a T1 growth not to be ethical.

Future improvement of survival rates and quality of life are
expected from various new approaches. The effect of adjuvant Flagyl
is being assessed in a randomised prospective trial when a full
course of external irradiation is being given or if preoperative
irradiation followed by cystectomy is the method of treatment.
Intracavitary application of chemotherapeutic agents may improve
the prognosis in patients with miltiple superficial primary growths
or in those with a solitary T1 growth. CT scan and ultrasound might

add to the information about the primary and the lymph nodes and
offer the opportunity to adapt treatment to these findings.
Meticulous prospective collection of all data must eventually show
whether this additional burden on the patient is justified by better
results.

REFERENCES

1.   U.I.C.C., T.N.M. Classification of Malignant Tumours, Geneva
     (1974).

2.   B. Van der Werf-Messing, Carcinoma vesicae urinariae treated
     at the Rotterdam Radiotherapy Institute, Archivum Urologicum
     8: 9 (1977).

3.   B. Van der Werf-Messing, Cancer of the urinary bladder treated
     by interstitial radium implant, Int. J. Radiation Oncology
     Biol. Phys. 4: 373 (1978).

4.   B. Van der Werf-Messing, Preoperative irradiation followed by
     cystectomy to treat carcinoma of the urinary bladder category
     T3NX,0-4MO, Int. J. Radiation Oncology Biol. Phys. 5: 394 (1979).

5.   B. Van der Werf-Messing, W.M. Star, and R.S. Menon, Carcinoma
     of the urinary bladder category T3NXMO treated by the combin-
     ation of radium implant and external irradiation. A preliminary
     Report. Int. J. Radiation Oncology Biol. Phys. (in press)

CHEMOTHERAPY

CHEMOTHERAPY FOR URINARY BLADDER CANCER:

DEVELOPMENTS, TRENDS, AND FUTURE PERSPECTIVES

G H JACOBI

Johannes Gutenberg-Universität
Mainz
West Germany

INTRODUCTION

The role of chemotherapy in the management of transitional bladder tumors can conveniently be considered under two principal headings - topical (intracavitary) and sytemic chemotherapy, as the indications for these modalities are distinctly different. The intent of topical administration of cytoxic agents may be (1) prophylactic to prevent recurrences or new occurrences after TUR; (2) curative to clear the bladder of extensive non-resectable multifocal disease, or to control carcinoma in situ.

Consequently, the indication for topical chemotherapy is, in itself, limited to superficial lesions. In cases of deeply infiltrating carcinoma in which cure can be achieved most rapidly by radical surgery, systemic chemotherapy may form an integrating adjuvant approach with curative intent to achieve downstaging of the tumor when given preoperatively, or to lower seeding from node metastases when given postoperatively. What remains is the most disappointing indication for systemic chemotherapy, i.e. palliative chemotherapy for far advanced cases with widespread tumor burden with the goals of improvement of quality of life and eventually even prolongation of survival.

In this regard, the report by Prout and Marshall (19) which states that patients with untreated bladder carcinoma of all stages survive on an average no longer than 11 - 18 months is a challenge.

Where do we stand in the 1980s with these tools of treatment? In the past two decades, Urologists have learned from their sometimes disappointing results with superficial papillary tumors

and with the potentially lethal types of cancer of the bladder that
the traditional surgical approach should ideally be supplemented by
other forms of treatment.   Three recent developments are likely to
influence attitudes quite markedly (1,2):-

1.   Urologists have adopted some of the attitudes of their colleagues
in medical oncology and have started to incorporate cytotoxic agents
in their therapy protocols.

2.   Medical Oncologists have recognised the poor outlook for the
patient with metastatic bladder cancer and have shown increasing
enthusiasm for phase I and II studies in patients with this disease.

3.   Local, regional and international cooperative groups have been
established including Urological surgeons, Medical Oncologists,
Statisticians and Pathologists to investigate the problems presented.

Although the individual doctor may suggest and promote new
treatments, the evaluation of treatments of potential benefit in such
a way that interpretable, reproducible and patient-orientated results
emerge and give valid guidelines for the future depends on several
factors including:-

1.   Laboratory investigations on the activity and tumor-orientated
properties of single agents or combinations of cytoxic drugs (6,9,
21,22).

2.   Multicenter cooperative studies to allow the recuitment of
large numbers of patients.

3.   Careful staging and grading of the tumor in all patients.

4.   Inderdisciplinary cooperation (24).

5.   Proper statistical control including randomisation, stratification where appropriate and statistical evaluation of all results
(24).

6.   Standardization of response criteria.

7.   Development and investigation of prognostic parameters such as
specific red cell adherence (SRCA) reaction and follow up cytology
(3,13).

Not all of these goals have yet been realised, but a number of
scientists, urological institutions and other organisations who are
actively participating in the development of chemotherapy in bladder
cancer should, however, be mentioned briefly.

In Europe the EORTC has developed protocols for intravesical and systemic administration of chemotherapeutic agents. On the basis of multicentric cooperative Phase II studies and Phase III trials, a number of results have been obtained (7,18,20,24). Also, the WHO has instituted a Collaborative Centre for Research and Treatment of Urinary Bladder Cancer at the Radiumhemmet, Karolinska Hospital in Stockholm. This institution has made valuable contributions by organising workshops, by experimental research programs and by clinical trials (4,5,6,22).

In the United Stages the National Bladder Cancer Collaborative Group is undertaking several randomised multicenter trials (16).

In addition, a number of individual investigators and institutions have, for years, made significant contributions including, among others, the Institute of Urology in London (17), the Memorial Sloan-Kettering Cancer Center in New York (27), the Roswell Park Memorial Institute in Buffalo (15) and others (3,8-13,19,21-23,25).

In the following, some factors of significance as well as the experimental and clinical basis for chemotherapy will briefly be summarised.

INTRACAVITARY CHEMOTHERAPY AND CHEMOPROPHYLAXIS

The potential advantage of applying a high concentration of a cytoxic agent directly to the site of tumor growth while minimising systemic exposure of other organs to the agent has been widely exploited in the past. Since the beginning of the century, a variety of toxic agents, heavy metals, astringents, radioactive solutions, antimetabolites, alkylating agents, antineoplastic antibiotics and other substances have been instilled into the bladder for cancer treatment. The development and use of these substances has been well reviewed in recent years (9,18,23).

Since electroresection and fulguration was always considered the treatment of choice, instillation therapy, particularly Thiotepa, was most often used to prevent recurrences. When talking about the pronounced tendency of superficial papillary urothelial bladder tumors to rapid recurrence (multiplicity "in time" and "in space") one must, particularly when dealing with retrospectively evaluated results, face the problem of true recurrence, new occurence, and residual tumor left behind at TUR (23). There is no doubt that some sort of carcinogenically mediated panurothelial disease (14) is involved in the chronic character of the condition. There is, however, clear-cut evidence that some iatrogenic factor, probably tumor implantation on the urothelium traumatised by heat, is a factor in propagation (8,18,22,23). At our Institution, intracavitary chemotherapy for local tumor control is extremely rare (25) and is only considered as palliation if the extent of "papillomatosis" does not allow extensive TUR. The benefits in terms of

tumor disappearance are inconsistent and hard to define; also we do
not know the exact stage and grade of the lesion we are treating and
we run the risk of "treating" the tip of an iceberg!

Therapeutic effects are often classified as "complete" or
"partial regression" or even "objective remission". These are mis-
leading as they cannot be standardised and are not interpretable for
comparative purposes.

In the treatment of patients with carcinoma in situ, however,
the situation is quite different. This lesion, which most Urologists
would, if multi-focal and symptomatic, consider as an indication for
radical surgery, is a condition which can be controlled by intravesical chemotherapy (12). Repeated urinary cytology and punch biopsy
are valuable tools in monitoring these patients' follow-up, in order
to evaluate the response to therapy and to determine the moment when
surgical treatment can no longer be postponed.

The true role for intracavitary administration of cytotoxic
agents, however, remains topical chemoprophylaxis. The goal of such
treatment is to reduce the recurrence rate by extending the disease-
free interval (delay of recurrence) and by inhibiting progression of
tumor stage and grade. Certain factors should be considered in the
design of future phase III trials:-

1.   The bladder must be cleared of all visible tumors by TUR and
the presence or absence of additional carcinoma in situ should be
verified by random biopsies (3,9,18,23,25).

2.   The substance must have been demonstrated to be active in animal
experiments and in human phase II studies (21-23).

3.   The cytotoxic agent should show good penetration into the urothelium without significant systemic absorption (9,18).

4.   The incidence of local and systemic toxicity should be low.

5.   Treatment must be possible on an outpatient basis.

6.   The agent should be free of carcinogenic activity.

7.   There should be an acceptable cost-versus-benefit relationship.

While requirements nos. 1 - 5 seem to be at least partially
fulfilled in a number of studies (4,5,8-10,18,20,23,26), the answers
to topics nos. 6 and 7 cannot as yet be determined.

Other significant questions, as outlined in C.C. Schulman's
paper in this volume, remain to be answered by future trials, such
as the time of initiation of instillation therapy (pre-, intra-

operatively, immediately after TUR, or after re-epithelisation),
duration of time the drug is to be kept in the bladder, the time
intervals between each instillation (? days, ? weeks), the dose per
instillation and the overall length of treatment (? 6 months, ? 1
year, ? indefinitely). Another problem only occasionally faced, is
the proper selection of patients including whether instillation
should be advised after the first tumor or only after several
recurrences. Tests which can select patients with a high risk of
recurring and progressing tumors, as for example, the SRCA- reaction
might in the future prove to be valuable tools in this regard (13).

Staquet (24) has already emphasised the need for randomised
trials to solve these problems. The trials must be completed before
this therapy can be recommended for routine use if one is to minimise
toxicity and obtain the greatest benefit from this therapy, which
may prove to be expensive.

SYSTEMIC CHEMOTHERAPY

As outlined before, this form of treatment has largely been
used for palliation in cases of locally extensive, so-called loco-
regional disease or in cases with widespread dissemination. A
dilemma for the therapist remains, however, the question of rigid
response criteria as outlined by Yagoda in this volume. For example,
it is hard to define "at least 50% reduction in size of all measurable tumor lesions" if the primary involves several structures in
the true pelvis. Thus, measurable distant metastases, so called
indicator lesions, are used . We must, however, be careful not to
forget the patients' individual requirements, namely improvement of
quality of life - not primarily the shrinkage of a pulmonary or
osseous cancer deposit - whilst hunting for a measurable lesion.
We must also consider whether it is ethical to involve preterminal
cancer patients in repeated extensive, sometimes invasive, work-ups
to fulfil the requirements of a study protocol. We must also avoid
the risk of seeing such patients as "randomised cases" rather than
as individuals needing patient-orientated tumor care. At the moment
bladder cancer chemotherapy prolongs life for only a few months, a
point which clearly demonstrates the great responsibility we all
have to keep in mind.

Another question in the issue is adjunctive chemotherapy, in
which the drugs are given with potentially curative intent. Since
we fail to salvage some 50 - 70% of patients with deeply infiltrating loco-regional tumors solely by radical surgical means, this
group might be expected to benefit greatly from adjunctive chemotherapy. If such treatment proves to be indicated, we must decide
whether it should be started before or after radical cystectomy,
whether patients without nodal involvement should be included or
excluded, whether preoperative chemotherapy is more effective than
radiotherapy in terms of tumor downstaging, whether there are

reasons to expect higher postoperative morbidity after preoperative
chemotherapy, whether preoperative low-dose irradiation will limit
the use of postoperative chemotherapy and whether we can hope for
less nephrotic analogs of effective agents for patients with cancer-
mediated impairment of renal function (21).

These and other questions are still open, emphasising again
the necessity for randomised controlled trials and an awareness of
the difficulties in evaluating such studies in which surgical
procedures, where the standardisation of procedures between centres
are inevitably limited, are included.

From this brief summary it seems clear that all involved in
the chemotherapy of patients with bladder cancer will need to
harness their energies in a disciplined and coordinated manner and
may well profit from a continuing awareness of the progress being
achieved by this form of therapy in the control of other malignant
diseases.

REFERENCES

1.   L.F. Arduino, Chemotherapy of carcinoma of the bladder, in:
     "Benign and Malignant Tumors of the Urinary Bladder,"
     E. Maltry, ed, Hans Huber Publ., Bern-Stuttgart-Vienna,
     pp 167 - 188 (1971).
2.   S.K. Carter, The chemotherapy of bladder cancer, in: "Chemo-
     therapy of Urogenital Tumors," G.P. Murphy and A. Mittelman,
     eds., Charles C. Thomas Publ., Springfield, pp 105 - 127 (1975).
3.   L. Denis, P. Nowé, and G. Declercq, Diagnostic contribution of
     bladder washing and multiple biopsies in bladder cancer, Eur.
     Urol. 6: 137 (1980).
4.   F. Edsmyr and L. Anderson, Chemotherapy in bladder carcinoma,
     Urol. Res. 6: 263 (1978).
5.   F. Edsmyr, T. Berlin, F. Boman, M. Duchek, P.L. Esposti,
     H. Gustafsson, H. Wijkström, and L.G. Collste, Intravesical
     therapy with adriamycin in patients with superficial tumors,
     Eur. Urol. 6: 132 (1980).
6.   S. Eksborg, S.-O. Nilsson, and F. Edsmyr, Intravesical instil-
     lation of adriamycin^R, A model for standardization of the
     chemotherapy, Eur. Urol. 6: 218 (1980).
7.   EORTC Urological Group B, The treatment of advanced carcinoma
     of the bladder with a combination of adriamycin and 5-fluor-
     ouracil, Eur. Urol. 3: 276 (1977).
8.   G.H. Jacobi, K.H. Kurth, K.F. Klippel, and R. Hohenfellner,
     On the biological behaviour of T1-transitional cell tumors of
     the urinary bladder and initial results of the prophylactic use
     of topical adriamycin under controlled and randomised con-
     ditions, in: "Diagnostics and Treatment of Superficial Urinary
     Bladder Tumors, WHO Collaborating Centre for Research and
     Treatment of Urinary Bladder Cancer," Montedison Lakemedel,
     Stockholm, pp 83 - 94 (1979).

9. G.H. Jacobi and K.H. Kurth, Studies on the intravesical action of topically administered G^3H-doxorubicin hydrochloride in men: plasma uptake and tumor penetration, J. Urol. 124: 34 (1980).

10. G.H. Jacobi, Institute of Urology Workshop: New Approaches to Treatment of Superficial and Invasive Bladder Carcinoma, London, (in press) 1979.

11. G. Jakse and F. Hofstädter, Further experiences with the specific red cell adherence test (SRCA) in bladder cancer. A histological and cytological study, Eur. Urol. 4: 356 (1978).

12. G. Jakse and F. Hofstädter, Intravesical doxorubicin hydrochloride in the management of carcinoma in situ of the bladder, A preliminary report. Eur. Urol. 6: 103 (1980).

13. G. Jakse, The effects of intravesical Adriamycin instillations for control of carcinoma in situ, mode of action, ultrastructure changes and clinical results, J. Urol (in press).

14. T. Kakizoe, F. Fujita, T. Murase, K. Matsumoto, and K. Kishi, Transitional cell carcinoma of the bladder in patients with renal pelvic and ureteral cancer, J. Urol. 124: 17 (1980).

15. C.E. Merrin, Institute of Urology Workshop: New Approaches to Treatment of Superficial and Invasive Bladder Carcinoma, London, 1979 (in press).

16. National Bladder Cancer Collaborative Group A, Surveillance, initial assessment and subsequent progress of patients with superficial bladder cancer in a prospective longitudinal study, Cancer Res. 37: 2907 (1977).

17. T. Oliver, Institute of Urology Workshop: New Approaches to Treatment of Superficial and Invasive Bladder Carcinoma, London, 1979 (in press).

18. M. Pavone-Macaluso, Intravesical treatment of superficial (T1) urinary bladder tumors, A review of a 15-year experience, in: "Diagnostics and Treatment of Superficial Urinary Bladder Tumors, WHO Collaborating Centre for Research and Treatment of Urinary Bladder Cancer," Montedison Lakemedel, Stockholm, pp 21 - 36 (1979).

19. G.R. Prout and V.T. Marshall, The prognosis with untreated bladder tumors, Cancer 9: 551 (1956).

20. C.C. Schulman, M. Rozencweig, M. Staquet, Y. Kenis, and R. Sylvester, EORTC randomised trial for the adjuvant therapy of T1 bladder carcinoma, Eur. Urol. 2: 271 (1976).

21. M.S. Soloway and C.E. Cox, Effect of platinum analogues and combination chemotherapy on murine bladder cancer, Trans. Amer. Ass. Genito-Urinary Surg. 71: 8 (1979).

22. M.S. Soloway and S. Masters, Urothelial susceptibility to tumor cell implantation, Cancer 46: 1158 (1980).

23. M.S. Soloway, Rationale for inensive intravesical chemotherapy for superficial bladder cancer, J. Urol. 123: 461 (1980).

24. M. Staquet, The randomised clinical trial: A prerequisite for rational therapy, Eur. Urol. 2: 265 (1976).

25. J.W. Thüroff and G.H. Jacobi, Therapy, follow-up treatment and
     prophylaxis of urinary bladder carcinoma, <u>Onkologie</u> 3: 248
     (1980).
26. WHO Collaborating Centre for Research and Treatment of Urinary
     Bladder Cancer, Diagnostics and Treatment of Superficial
     Urinary Bladder Tumors, Montedison Lakemedel, Stockholm (1979).
27. A. Yagoda, Phase II trials in bladder cancer at Memorial Sloan-
     Kettering Cancer Center, 1975 - 1978, <u>in</u>: "Cancer of the Genito-
     urinary Tract," D.E. Johnson and M.L. Samuels, eds., Raven Press,
     New York, pp 107 - 119 (1979).

INTRAVESICAL CHEMOTHERAPY FOR SUPERFICIAL BLADDER TUMORS

C C SCHULMAN

Hôpital Erasme
Bruxelles
Belgium

INTRODUCTION

Superficial bladder tumors (T1, pT1 of the TNM classification (UICC, 1974) or Jewett Stage 0 and A) are usually treated by trans-urethral resection (TUR). However, recurrence of the tumor after complete resection occurs in about 60% of the patients (8, 10, 21, 22, 28) with a significant percentage of these recurrences showing a higher degree of malignancy (10, 22). In 10% of the cases the tumor progresses to invasive carcinoma (8) and the 5-year survival rate following TUR is about 62% (8, 18, 28). Most of these recurrent tumors will occur within 6 to 12 months.

Several factors are of prognostic importance in the prediction of recurrences including the number of tumors at the time of diagnosis and first treatment; the size of the tumor (100% recurrences if tumor larger than 4 cm in Mayo Clinic series); and the frequency of recurrences. Two different concepts are considered to explain the high incidence of recurrences, although both mechanisms may occur together.

EPITHELIAL DISEASE

The diffuse nature of the epithelial hyperplasia, dysplasia and neoplastic change is well documented. Multiple mucosal biopsies from either random or pre-selected endoscopically normal areas in patients with bladder tumor have shown a high incidence of atypia, carcinoma in situ and even carcinoma in these cystoscopically normal areas (6, 13, 15, 20). Follow-up revealed a much higher incidence of bladder cancer in patients with abnormalities in these biopsies than in those without such findings (38% against 16%) (13).

101

This follow-up suggests that some of these cellular abnormalities
progress to neoplasia and that mucosal alteration is responsible
for most of the subsequent tumors that develop after resection of a
superficial bladder tumor. These tumoral growths might better be
called new occurrences rather than recurrences since they do not
represent a regrowth of the original neoplasm (22).

Industrial carcinogens (naphthylamine, benzidine, 4-amino-
diphenyl) and also cigarettes are epidemiologic factors of importance. They can induce tumors or act as promotors. Chronic urinary
tract infection and stones have also been considered to be involved
in the development of bladder tumors (11).

TUMOR IMPLANTATION

The concept of implantation of bladder tumor was first made
by Albarran and Imbert in 1903 (1). Since that time several reports
have emphasized that the areas traumatized during TUR or fulguration
are the most likely to allow implantation of neoplastic cells and
subsequent recurrences (23, 24, 26).

The concept is further supported by the study of Burnand et al.
(3) who instilled Thiotepa immediately after tumor resection in order
to destroy neoplastic cells floating free within the bladder. They
compared the results with those obtained in a control group. There
was a significant diminution of the recurrences in the group receiving Thiotepa suggesting that implanting tumor cells were destroyed
in those patients who remained free of recurrent tumors.

Most likely implantation and new occurrences are involved in the
recurrence of superficial bladder tumor. The disease might represent
a different potential evolution in each patient.

The therapeutic implications of these concepts are obvious.
Those who favour the idea of a diffuse urothelial disease advocate
repeated and prolonged instillation of chemotherapeutic agents.
People who are in favour of the tumor implantation theory advocate
early, immediate instillation of drugs into the bladder to destroy
the remaining floating neoplastic cells. Since it is not possible
to prove or disprove either of these concepts at the present time it
is wiser to consider that both theories are correct and that multifocal urothelial disease and implantation of tumor cells may occur
separately or simultaneously.

Thus, a combined therapeutic approach would seem advisable -
by early instillation of chemotherapeutic agents in the bladder
with repeated instillations at regular intervals for at least one
year. If, despite this regimen a patient continues to develop
multiple recurrences, he must be considered as having a potential
risk of uncontrollable urothelial disease with the risk of

progression to a more malignant tumor and more aggressive and
radical treatment should be considered.

INDICATIONS FOR LOCAL CHEMOTHERAPY

Two main purposes might be considered for the use of intravesical chemotherapy in bladder tumors: treatment and
prophylaxis.

Therapy

Drugs have been instilled in the bladder to destroy multiple
papillary tumors (16, 25). The objective followed in this
situation is to achieve total or partial regression of tumors.

Intravesical chemotherapy, mainly with Adriamycin, has been
advocated recently for the treatment of carcinoma in situ (2, 5).
This treatment was initiated to achieve the disappearance of
neoplastic cells followed by cytological examination. Promising
results have been achieved (5).

Prophylaxis

The main indication for intravesical chemotherapy in superficial bladder tumors is prophylactic, to reduce the recurrence
of tumors after their removal by TUR, fulguration or open surgery.
The main objectives are a reduction of the recurrence rate (number-
size-stage of tumors) and an increase of the disease-free interval
(21).

Several treatments adjuvant to TUR have been advocated in an
attempt to increase the survival rate, the disease-free interval
and to reduce the recurrence rate. Periodic instillation of
Thiotepa, a cytotoxic alkylating agent, has been used for more than
15 years, both for prophylaxis and for the treatment of recurrent
T1 bladder tumors, but controversy still continues regarding the
precise indications for its use (8, 22, 25, 27). Staquet (20) has
recently reviewed nine non-randomized studies with intravesical
Thiotepa and found a success rate ranging from 24% to 100% (4).

Several other drugs have been employed for local chemotherapy
often with conflicting results including thiotepa (3, 4, 9, 25, 27);
doxorubicin (adriamycin) (2, 5); mitomycin C (12); epodyl (14, 19);
epipodophyllotoxin (VM 26) (17); and cis-platinum. Other compounds
have been studied in the past but are no longer in use because of
lack of effectiveness or toxicity. The results of studies on
several of the potentially active drugs have recently been reviewed
by Soloway (22).

In the choice of a drug for intravesical chemotherapy

stringent criteria should be met. The drug must be active, have
no systemic toxicity, have a low absorption through the bladder
wall with few or no local effects, demonstrate good penetration into
the bladder wall and should not be mutagenic. Few drugs, if any,
comply with these requirements.

TREATMENT REGIMEN

Several questions remain to be answered before the ideal
treatment regimen can be designed. Some of these problems can be
briefly discussed, including:-

Timing

Should the first instillation be given early after TUR or
delayed? Early chemotherapy is often advocated to prevent tumor
implantation but others object for fear of a higher incidence of
local or even systemic effects from increased absorption into and
through the bladder wall via the traumatized areas of bladder
mucosa.

Length of treatment

Should the intravesical administration of drugs be given in a
single dose or should prolonged treatment be advocated? The
concept of urothelial disease favours prolonged treatment.

Duration of instillation

The time of contact between the instilled drug and the bladder
mucosa is usually 60 minutes. This is, however, quite an empirical
approach and may need to be varied according to the drug used and to
its concentration.

Frequency of instillations

Should the drug be instilled at short intervals soon after
TUR or should a period of one week, or perhaps one month, be allowed
between instillations?

Dose

The optimal dose to be employed for the various drugs is not
yet determined. The total dose as well as the dose/time relationship is also of importance. Recently standardization of treatment
for each patient has been advocated based on the concentration
rather than on the dose at which the drug is used. It is suggested
that the bladder capacity should be measured first and a volume
instilled equal to bladder capacity minus 50 ml so that the con-

centration remains constant for each patient whereas the volume and dose of drugs vary with each patient.

This concept also relies on the assumption that maximal distention of the bladder is desirable in order to obtain a close contact between the drug and the whole surface of the bladder mucosa. This is not proved and other authors prefer to use a small volume to achieve a higher concentration of the drug and a prolonged contact time.

EORTC COOPERATIVE STUDY (EORTC Protocol 30751)

The Urological Group of the EORTC, a multi-institutional cooperative group, has performed a randomized clinical trial designed to compare, after TUR alone or TUR followed by bladder instillation of thiotepa or VM 26 (21) in patients with category T1 bladder cancer:-

  i. the disease-free interval;
 ii. the recurrence rate;
iii. the number of patients with increase in tumor stage.

Drug instillation was initiated one month post-operatively and subsequent treatment was administered weekly for 4 weeks and then monthly for one year. Summarized analysis of the results have shown that although there was no difference among the groups regarding the time of first recurrence, thiotepa significantly reduced the recurrence rate as compared to VM 26 or no treatment. When adjusting by stratification for primary or recurrent patients the results remained the same (Tables 1, 2, 3).

This study, performed on a large number of patients, allowed a study of the importance of several variables as factors playing a role in the recurrence of tumors.

Two logistic models have been tried, one considering the recurrence rate as the number of recurrences divided by the number of cystoscopies and the second where the recurrence rate was calculated as the number of recurrences divided by the number of months to follow-up. Both models yielded similar results and have shown that, of the variables tested, those of greatest relevance were, in order of importance:-

   i.   the number of tumors;
  ii.   the number of previous recurrences (before entering the
        study;
 iii.   the size of the tumor;
  iv.   treatment with thiotepa.

Therefore the profile of the patient with the least chance of

TABLE 1

EORTC Protocol 30751

Recurrences by Treatment (All Patients)

	Thiotepa	VM 26	No Treatment	Total
No of patients randomized	122	124	124	370
No of patients with follow-up	106	106	103	315
No of patients with recurrences	65	77	71	213
Per cent with recurrences	61.3	72.6	68.9	67.6
Total no of recurrences	105	109	140	354
Total months of follow-up	1863	1590	1543	4996
Recurrence rate/100 patient months	5.64	6.86	9.07	7.09

TABLE 2

EORTC Protocol 30751

Recurrences by Treatment (Primary patients)

	Thiotepa	VM 26	No Treatment	Total
No of patients randomized	78	75	78	231
No of patients with follow-up	68	65	60	193
No of patients with recurrences	38	42	35	115
Per cent with recurrences	55.9	64.6	58.3	59.6
Total no of recurrences	51	61	64	176
Total months of follow-up	1242	1068	963	3273
Recurrence rate/100 patient months	4.11	5.71	6.45	5.38

TABLE 3

EORTC Protocol 30751

Recurrences by Treatment (Recurrent patients)

	Thiotepa	VM 26	No Treatment	Total
No of patients randomized	45	48	46	139
No of patients with follow-up	38	41	43	122
No of patients with recurrences	27	35	36	98
Per cent with recurrences	71.1	85.4	83.7	80.3
Total no of recurrences	54	48	76	178
Total months of follow-up	620	522	580	1722
Recurrence rate/100 patient months	8.71	9.20	13.10	10.34

recurrence would be: a solitary tumor at TUR which was a primary lesion, less than or equal to 2 cms (and treated with thiotepa). The patient with the worst prognosis would have 3 or more tumors at TUR, more than 2 recurrences/year before randomization, the largest tumor 3 or more cms in size (and not treated with thiotepa).

BELGIAN MULTICENTER STUDY OF EARLY ADJUVANT INSTILLATION OF ADRIAMYCIN IN T1 BLADDER TUMORS

A multicenter study was recently performed in Belgium, involving 6 university or affiliated institutions in which Adriamycin (50 mg/50 ml) was administered intravesically within 24 hours after TUR for T1 bladder tumors. Instillation was repeated on the third and seventh day during the first week, weekly during the first month and then monthly for one year. Two main aspects were considered in analyzing the results - tolerance and prevention of recurrence (Table 4, 5).

A total of 110 patients were entered into this study. All were evaluable for tolerance. Of these, 23 patients (26.3%) presented with mild side effects and remained on treatment; in 3 of these patients the dose was halved in subsequent instillations. 24 patients presented with severe side effects and went off study (21.8%). One patient suffered a myocardial infarct 10 months after TUR and following 14 instillations. This was considered to be an incidental finding and not a toxic effect. Follow-up for recurrence over a period of one year was possible in 82 patients. Of these the initial tumor was primary in 23 patients and recurrent in 59 (Table 5). Of these 82 patients recurrences were seen in 32 (39%). Of the recurrences 27 were category T1 tumors while 5 patients developed invasive lesions. Among the 23 primary patients 19 were free of tumors while 4 had T1 recurrence (17.4%). Among 59 recurrent cases 28 presented with recurrences (47.4%).

TABLE 4

Belgian Multicenter Study of Early Adriamycin Instillation
in T1 Bladder Tumors
- Side effects in 110 evaluable patients

Local Side Effects

Still under Treatment	Treatment Stopped
29 (26.3%)	26 ⎰ Progression - 2 ⎱ Local toxicity - 24 (21.8%)

TABLE 5

Belgian Multicenter Study of Early Adriamycin Instillation
in T1 Bladder Tumors
Recurrences in 110 patients

(Primary tumors 33; Recurrent tumors 77)

Evaluable patients (one year follow-up) - 82	Primary Tumors - 23	Recurrent Tumors - 59
Recurrence during Therapy	4 - T1	28 ⟨ 23 (T1) / 5 > T1

The percentage recurrence rate in patients with primary and
recurrent tumors in this study using early Adriamycin instillation
compares favourably with the percentage of recurrences in the same
groups in the EORTC study in which thiotepa, VM 26 and a control
group were studied (Tables 1-3). It must be remembered however
that the period of follow-up is longer in the EORTC study and it
is hoped to add to this information with the current EORTC protocols
comparing intravesical thiotepa, adriamycin and epodyl.

REFERENCES

1.   J. Albarran and L. Imbert, "Les Tumeurs du Rein", Masson et Cie,
pp 452 - 459, Paris (1903).
2.   M.D. Banks, J.E. Pontes, R.M. Izbicki and J.M. Pierce Jr.,
Topical instillation of doxorubicin hydrochloride in the treatment
of recurring superficial transitional cell carcinoma of the bladder,
J. Urol. 118: 757 (1977).
3.   K.G. Burnand, P.J.R. Boyd, M.E. Mayo, K.E.D. Shuttleworth and
R.W. Lloyd-Davies, Single dose intravesical thiotepa as an adjuvant
to cystodiathermy in the treatment of transitional cell bladder
carcinoma, Brit. J. Urol. 48: 55 (1976).
4.   D. Byar and C. Blackard, Comparisons of placebo, pyridoxine and
topical thiotepa in preventing recurrence of Stage 1 bladder cancer,
Urol. 10: 556 (1977).
5.   F. Edsmyr, T. Berlin, J. Boman, M. Duchek, P.L. Esposti,
H. Gustafsson, H. Wijkström and L.G. Collste, Intravesical therapy
with Adriamycin in patients with superficial tumors, Eur. Urol. 6:
132 - 136 (1980).
6.   R.B. Eisenberg, R.B. Roth and M.H. Schweinsberg, Bladder tumors
and associated proliferative mucosal lesions, J. Urol. 84: 544
(1960).
7.   S. Eksborg, S.O. Nilsson and F. Edsmyr, Intravesical instillation of Adriamycin. A model for standardization of the chemotherapy,
Eur. Urol. 6: 218 (1980).

8. L.F. Greene, K.A. Hanash and G.M. Farrow, Benign papilloma or papillary carcinoma of the bladder? J. Urol. 110: 205 (1973).
9. H.C. Jones and J. Swinney, Thiotepa in the treatment of tumors of the bladder, Lancet 2: 615 (1961).
10. R.I Lerman, R.V. Hutter and W.F. Whitmore Jr., Papilloma of the urinary bladder, Cancer 25: 333 (1970).
11. A.B. Miller, The etiology of bladder cancer from the epidemiological viewpoint, Cancer Res. 37: 2939 (1977).
12. T. Mishina, K. Oda, S. Murata, H. Ooe, Y. Mori and T. Takahashi, Mitomycin C bladder instillation therapy for bladder tumors, J. Urol. 114 : 217 (1975).
13. W.M. Murphy, G.K. Nagy, M.D. Rao, M.S. Soloway, G.C. Parija, C.E. Cox and G.H. Friedell, Normal urothelium in patients with bladder cancer, Cancer 44: 1050 (1979).
14. H.V. Nielsen and E. Thybo, Epodyl treatment of bladder tumors, Scan. J. Urol. Nephrol. 13: 59 (1979).
15. B.H. Page, V.B. Levison and M.P. Curwen, The site of recurrence of non-infiltrating bladder tumors, Brit. J. Urol. 50: 237 (1978).
16. M. Pavone-Macaluso, Chemotherapy of vesical and prostatic tumors, Brit. J. Urol. 43: 701 (1971).
17. M. Pavone-Macaluso, Preliminary evaluation of VM 26: a new epipodophyllotoxin derivative in the treatment of urogenital tumors, Eur. Urol. 1: 53 (1975).
18. L.N. Pyrah, F.P. Raper and G.M. Thomas, Report of a follow-up of papillary tumors of the bladder, Brit. J. Urol. 36: 14 (1964).
19. P.R. Riddle, The management of superficial bladder tumors with intravesical epodyl, Brit. J. Urol. 45: 84 (1973).
20. R.O.K. Schade and J. Swinney, The association of urothelial atypism with neoplasia: its importance in treatment and prognosis, J. Urol. 109: 619 (1973).
21. C. Schulman, M. Rozencweig, M. Staquet, Y. Kenis and R. Sylvester, EORTC randomized trial for the adjuvant therapy of T1 bladder carcinoma, Eur. Urol. 2: 271 (1976).
22. M. Soloway, Rationale for intensive intravesical chemotherapy for superficial bladder cancer, J. Urol. 123: 461 (1980).
23. M.S. Soloway, W. Murphy, M.K. Rao and C. Cox, Serial multiple-site biopsies in patients with bladder cancer, J. Urol. 120: 57 (1978).
24. M.S. Soloway and S. Masters, Implantation of transitional tumor cells on the cauterized murine urothelial surface, Proc. Amer. Ass. Cancer Res. 20: 256 (1979).
25. R.J. Veenema, A.L. Dean Jr., M. Roberts, B. Fingerhut, B.K. Chowdhury and H. Tarassoly, Bladder carcinoma treated by direct instillation of thiotepa, J. Urol. 88: 60 (1962).
26. A.C. Wallace and E.S. Hershfield, The experimental implantation of tumor cells in the urinary tract, Brit. J. Cancer 12: 622 (1958).
27. J.W. Wescott, The prophylactic use of thiotepa in transitional cell carcinoma of the bladder, J. Urol. 96: 913 (1966).
28. J.L. Williams, J.C. Hammonds and N. Saunders, T1 bladder tumors Brit. J. Urol. 49: 663 (1977).

PROGRESS IN THE CHEMOTHERAPEUTIC TREATMENT OF ADVANCED BLADDER

CANCER

A YAGODA

Memorial Sloan-Kettering Cancer Center
New York
U S A

The introduction of cisplatin in 1976 (35) in the treatment of patients with transitional cell carcinoma of the urothelial tract, i.e. renal pelvis, ureter, bladder, urethra and prostatic ducts, has led to a systematic evaluation of chemotherapeutic agents for advanced bladder cancer. Disease-orientated phase II trials, some utilizing strict patient selection and response criteria, have confirmed cisplatin's antitumor activity - 35% (27, 10, 39) and recently phase III prospectively randomized disease-orientated studies have been instituted. This paper will outline presently available data and discuss two recently completed trials at Memorial Sloan-Kettering Cancer Center which utilize methotrexate (38, 17) and vinblastine (1), each used singly.

Since the pattern of recurrence in patients with bladder cancer is frequently in the pelvis, intra-abdominally and loco-regionally, the accurate assessment of 'significant (> 50%) tumor reduction has been difficult (32). In an elegant study by Moertel et al (13) who used lucite balls placed under a mattress to simulate intra-abdominal lesions, repeated measurements of "tumor masses" by 16 experienced oncologists were relatively accurate. Changes in the size of bladder or pelvic masses by rectal examination, particularly after radiation and/or surgery, would also be fraught with such imprecision. Thus, bidimensionally measurable tumor masses are a prerequisite in phase II disease-orientated trials in bladder cancer for defining a clear end-point of response (32). In many instances it is appropriate for large scale phase III studies to utilize patients with only evaluable, uni-dimensional parameters, but phase II trials should continue to evaluate patients with objectively measurable bidimensional "indicator" lesions - pulmonary, nodal, cutaneous, subcutaneous and hepatic, pelvic and intra-abdominal masses which have

been found to be bidimensional on computerized transaxial tomography.
It should be recognized however, that no tumor has a homogenous cell
population and that recent evidence does suggest differences in
response to single agent therapy in disseminated sites such as pulmonary and nodal disease compared to intravesical (T2-4) lesions (20).
In order to effectively evaluate antitumor activity it might be more
useful to have separate trials for disseminated and intravesical
lesions and, whenever possible, reviews should not group all responses together.

Single Agents

Cisplatin has been employed in doses of 1.6 mg/kg, 70 mg/m^2,
75 mg/m^2 and 20 mg/m^2 for five consecutive days, every three to four
weeks.   The overall response rate in 162 cases is 35% with the 95%
confidence limits between 27 to 43% (Table 1).   Symptomatic improvement is often observed within the first 10 days, and objective tumor
regression can be noted in 7-21 days.   In only one instance has
tumor regression been noted to begin 35 days after initiation of
cisplatin therapy.   The median duration of response is 5-6 months,
and unmaintained remissions have persisted for 3-60 months.   A small
number of patients have remained in remission for 18 to 48+ months.
Nausea, vomiting, anorexia and nephrotoxicity have been persistent
problems with cisplatin administration and although adjuvant trials
have been initiated, long term therapy with cisplatin is generally
not accepted by patients.   Recently, Oliver (20), Herr (10) and
Soloway (28) have described patients who have shown evidence of local
relapse in spite of persistence of a systemic remission in nodal or
pulmonary sites.   After surgical resection such patients have remained in remission which suggests that cisplatin may be more effective
in the treatment of patients with disseminated disease than in those
with loco-regional disease (20).

Adriamycin generally has been administered in doses of 30, 45,
60, 75 and 90 mg/m^2.   While initial response rates were in the 35-
55% range, in over 185 cases the overall rate, when minor remissions
are excluded, is only 17% (34).   Responses are not as rapidly seen
as with cisplatin and generally require two to three doses, or three
to nine weeks.   The average duration of response is only three to
four months.   O'Bryan et al (19) have suggested a dose response
curve, and Yagoda et al (36) have noted a similar finding.

The Royal Marsden Hospital Group (9, 30) has evaluated methotrexate in three dosage schedules: 50 mg. or 100 mg. i.m. every two
weeks and 200 mg. i.m. with citrovorum factor rescue every one to
two weeks.   Of 50 patients, the majority of whom had loco-regional
T3 lesions which were assessed by bimanual palpation under anesthesia,
25-50% achieved objective tumor regression.   The response rate
appeared to be higher with the higher dosage schedule.   In that trial
a few patients did have disseminated disease and one patient

TABLE 1

Single Agent Trials in Bladder Cancer

Drug	No. Adeq.	% CR+PR
Cisplatin	162	35 (28-43)
Methotrexate	151	28 (21-35)
Adriamycin	183	17 (12-22)
AMSA	19	11
Bleomycin	58	5
Cyclophosphamide	98	31*
5-Fluorouracil	105	28*
Hexamethylmelamine	36	35**
Mitomycin C	42	13
Neocarcinostatin	19	5
PALA	18	0
VM-26	79	20
VP-16	18	0
Vinblastine	21	38 (20-60)
Yoshi 864	11	18

( ) = 95% confidence limits; *old studies, see text;
** most trials were in Bilharzial bladder cancer.

apparently achieved a complete remission for 14+ months.   Other
trials with methotrexate have been limited but recently Yagoda et
al (39) and Natale et al (17) have described a response rate of 27%
in 46 adequately treated patients of whom 42 had bidimensionally
measurable parameters.   The dose schedule was generally 0.5-1. -
1.5 mg/kg i.v. every week and all responses were evident within 21
days.   The median duration of remission was 4.5 months, and
responders appeared to have a longer survival than non-responders.
In addition, patients with a higher performance status (90-100
Karnofsky scale) and who had no prior chemotherapy (30% of patients)
achieved a higher response rate.   Of note, responses occurred in
28% of patients who had extensive prior chemotherapy.

     Other single agent trials have been limited (Table 1).   The
EORTC (21) has reported a 20% response rate in patients given the
podophyllin derivative VM-26, but of interest, no responses were
observed with another podophyllin derivative VP-16 (34, 18).   Limited trials at Memoral Sloan-Kettering Cancer Center (39) produced no
significant responses to the new acridine derivative m-AMSA

(4'-(9-acridinylamino)methanesulfon-m-anisidide) or with PALA
(phosphonoacetyl-l-aspartate) an aspartate transcarbamylase inhibitor.
The latter drug, when tested in the FANFT bladder carcinogen model,
was found to show moderate anti-tumor activity (28).   Other single
agent trials are listed in Table 1.   Neocarcinostatin has been
reported by Sakomoto et al (23) to exhibit significant anti-tumor
activity against intravesical lesions when administered intravenously
or intravesically but a trial in patients with disseminated disease
found only one response in 19 patients (16).   The data which is
available for cyclophosphamide and 5-fluorouracil represents usually
small numbers of cases from single trials which utilized older
criteria no longer acceptable today (34).

A recent trial (1) using vinblastine 0.1 mg/kg i.v. every week
has found significant anti-tumor activity in 8 of 22 adequately
treated patients of whom 15 have had extensive prior chemotherapy.
Eight (38%) responses were noted with tumor regression in pulmonary
lesions in five cases and in nodal sites in three.   The 95% confidence limits in this small series are 20-60%.   Many old and new agents
still require evaluation in disease-orientated phase II studies.

Combination Regimens

Adriamycin has been combined with cyclophosphamide and with
VM-26 without any evidence of synergism or an additive effect (Table
2) (33, 22).   There have been three reports (2, 3, 11) on the use
of 5-fluorouracil and adriamycin at a dose of 500 and 50 mg/m^2 i.v.
every three weeks, respectively.   While many cases were primarily
intravesical or loco-regional disease, some responses were described
in patients with disseminated disease (Table 2).   Further evaluation
of patients with bidimensionally measurable, disseminated disease
should be undertaken to confirm a potentially synergistic effect of
5-fluorouracil and adriamycin.   Williams et al (31) has added
cisplatin to the two drug combination, but the overall response rate
is approximately 45%.

Cisplatin has been combined with cyclophosphamide, adriamycin,
and cyclophosphamide and adriamycin.   Yagoda et al (37) described a
response rate of 44% and concluded that there was no additional
benefit from cyclophosphamide.   Narayana et al (14) recently reported only 2 of 10 patients responding to a similar drug combination.

Cisplatin 70 mg/m^2 and adriamycin 30-45-60 mg/m^2 induced remissions in 46% of patients in the Memorial Hospital series (34) and,
with a slightly different dosage schedule, only 36% of cases responded in a recently reported South West Oncology Group study (4).
The latter study randomized adriamycin vs. adriamycin and cisplatin
and achieved responses in 20 vs. 36% respectively.   In untreated
cases response increased to 45% (10/22 cases).   While the median
duration of response was seven months (34), slightly longer than that

TABLE 2

Combination Drug Trials in Bladder Cancer

Drugs	No. Adeq.	% CR+PR
Cisplatin + cyclophosphamide	45	38 (24-52)
Cisplatin + adriamycin	72	42 (30-53)
Cisplatin + adriamycin + 5-fluorouracil	44	41 (26-55)
Cisplatin + adriamycin + cyclophosphamide	94	41 (31-50)
Adriamycin + cyclophosphamide	39	18 (6-30)
Adriamycin + 5-fluouracil	103	39 (29-48)
Adriamycin + VM-26	27	19

( ) = 95% confidence limits.

achieved with cisplatin singly, the overall response rate could be attributed statistically to cisplatin alone (within the 95% confidence limits).

Cisplatin, adriamcyin and cyclophosphamide have been administered in various doses and schedules (34). In the Memorial Hospital series (34) cisplatin was given at a dose of $70 mg/m^2$ day 1, cyclophosphamide 250 mgs/m^2 day 2, and adriamycin 45 mg/m^2 day 3. This sequential regimen was based upon possible synergism in the FANFT tumor model when the dose of adriamycin was delayed 48-72 hours after cisplatin (28). In the "CISCA" protocol adriamycin 50 mg/m^2, cyclophosphamide 500 mg/m^2 were given on day 1, and cisplatin on day 2 at a dose of 100 mg/m^2. Courses were repeated every three to four weeks. Initially (29), 10 of 12 adequately treated patients had responded to the CISCA regimen, but two recent updates of the data has shown a response rate of 41% and 50% in 50 patients (24, 25). The overall duration of complete remission was five to seven months. Oliver (20) recently reported on 3 of 10 patients who responded but all remissions were in intravesical lesions. Again, the overall response rate to the three drug combination could be attributed to cisplatin alone.

Additional prospectively randomized trials are comparing cisplatin vs. cisplatin and cyclophosphamide, and cisplatin vs. cisplatin vs. adriamycin. The results of such studies should determine if there is any benefit from combination cisplatin regimens above that which could be expected with cisplatin alone. There is no

evidence so far, that any cisplatin combinations are clinically
synergistic.

Conclusion

Bladder cancer - the transitional cell variety - is a chemo-
therapeutically responsive tumor.   Cisplatin and adriamycin are
active as single agents.   In addition, some anti-tumor effect has
been shown with VM-26, vinblastine, mitomycin C and possibly with
5-fluorouracil and cyclophosphamide.   Cisplatin containing regimens
doe not appear to be any more effective than cisplatin alone and
adriamycin plus 5-fluorouracil needs further evaluation.   Future
trials might consider combinations of cisplatin and vinblastine and
methotrexate - unfortunately, cisplatin is nephrotoxic and methotrexate requires good renal function.   Many other single agents have
not been adequately evaluated.   In Bilharzial bladder cancer cisplatin, methotrexate and VM-26 are inactive, while hexamethylmelamine
- an agent which has not undergone extensive evaluation in transitional cell carcinoma - produces a 38% response rate (5, 6, 7, 8).

Since agents are available which induce reponses in 25-33%
of cases, adjuvant chemotherapy trials have been initiated and results of such studies will be of major interest.   Methotrexate is
another agent which should be considered for adjuvant studies.
Patients who have stage D or Pl-4 disease, in spite of pre-operative
irradiation and radical cystectomy, have a poor prognosis.   A recent
study at Memorial Hospital in 134 cases revealed that the five-year
survival after radical cystectomy was 7% and that 50% expired within
9-10 months (26).   The only group who did slightly better were those
who had microscopic disease in only one lymph node;   median survival
in 30 cases was 22 months.   Obviously, patients with N1 disease
require systemic chemotherapy since at least 50% who die have evidence
of disseminated disease (26, 12).   Thus, while loco-regional control
is relatively good, chemotherapy would be required to control unsus-
pected metastases.   Chemotherapy trials have been initiated in such
patients and one would expect clinical benefit evidenced by increased
survival with an aggressive chemotherapeutic approach.

Supported in part by Public Health Service grant CA-05826 and
contract NO 1-CM-57043 (Division of Cancer Treatment) from the
National Cancer Institute, National Institutes of Health, Department
of Health, Education and Welfare and donations from the Solid Tumor
Service Fund and from Mr Aaron Miller.

REFERENCES

1. M. Blumenreich, A. Yagoda, R.C. Watson and B. Needles, Phase II
    Trial of Vinblastine Sulfate in Bladder Cancer, Amer. Soc. Clin.
    Oncol. Abstr. (1981), in press.
2. R.J. Cross, R.W. Glashan, C.S. Humphrey, M.R.G. Robinson,
    P.H. Smith and R.E. Williams, Treatment of Advanced Bladder
    Cancer with Adriamycin and 5 Fluorouracil, Brit. J. Urol. 48:
    609 (1976).
3. EORTC, The Treatment of Advanced Carcinoma of the Bladder with
    a Combination of Adriamycin and 5 Fluorouracil, Eur. Urol. 3:
    276 (1977).
4. R. Gagliano, Adriamycin vs. Adriamycin plus Cisplatinum in
    Transitional Cell Bladder Carcinoma, Proc. Amer. Assoc. Cancer
    Res. 21: 347 (1980).
5. N.M. Gad-el-Mawla and J.L. Ziegler, Phase II Trial of Bleomycin
    in Bilharzial Bladder Cancer, Cancer Treat. Rep. 62: 1109 (1978a).
6. N.M. Gad-el-Mawla, R. Hamza, J. Cairns et al, Phase II Trial of
    Methotrexate in Carcinoma of the Bilharzial Bladder, Cancer
    Treat. Rep. 62: 1075 (1978b).
7. N.M. Gad-el-Mawla, F.M. Muggia, M.R. Hamza et al, Chemothera-
    peutic Management of Carcinoma of the Bilharzial Bladder: A
    Phase II Trial with Hexamethylmelamine and VM-26, Cancer Treat.
    Rep. 62: 993 (1978c).
8. N.M. Gad-el-Mawla, R. Hamza, E. Chevelen et al, Phase II Trial
    of Adriamycin in Carcinoma of the Bilharzial Bladder, Cancer
    Treat. Rep. 63: 227 (1979).
9. R.R. Hall, H.J.G. Bloom, J.E. Freeman et al, Methotrexate Treat-
    ment for Advanced Bladder Cancer, Brit. J. Urol. 46: 431 (1974).
10. H. Herr, Diamminedichloride Platinum II in the Treatment of
    Advanced Bladder Cancer, J. Urol. 123: 953 (1980).
11. S.B. Martinos and M. Al-Sarraf, Phase II Study of 5-Fluorouracil
    and Adriamycin in Transitional Cell Carcinoma of the Urinary
    Tract, Cancer Treat. Rep. 64: 161 (1980).
12. J.E. Montie, W.F. Whitmore, H.M. Grabstald and A. Yagoda,
    Management of Patients with Locally Unresectable Carcinoma of
    the Bladder, (in preparation).
13. C.G. Moertel and J.A. Hanley, The Effect of Measuring Error on
    the Results of Therapeutic Trials in Advanced Cancer, Cancer
    38: 388 (1976).
14. A.S. Narayana, S.A. Leoning and D.A. Culp, Chemotherapy for
    Advanced Carcinoma of the Bladder, Proc. Amer. Urol. Assoc. 75th
    Annual Meeting, 122: 104 (1980).
15. R.B. Natale, A. Yagoda and D. Molander, In Vitro and In Vivo
    Sensitivity of Human Bladder Carcinoma: Correlation with Phase
    II Trials of AMSA, PALA and Methotrexate, Proc. Amer. Assoc.
    Cancer Res. 21: 297 (1980a).
16. R.B. Natale, A. Yagoda, R.C. Watson et al, Phase II Trial of
    Neocarcinostatin in Patients with Prostatic and Bladder Cancer
    Cancer, 45: 2836 (1980b).

17. R.B. Natale, A. Yagoda, R.C. Watson et al, Methotrexate: An
     Active Drug in Bladder Cancer, Cancer (in press).
18. N.I. Nissen, T.F. Pajak, L.A. Leone et al, Clinical Trial of
     VP 16-213 (NSC 14150) i.v. Twice Weekly in Advanced Neoplastic
     Disease, Cancer 45: 232 (1980).
19. R.M. O'Bryan, L.H. Baker, J.E. Gottleib et al, Dose Response
     Evaluation of Adriamycin in Human Neoplasia, Cancer 39: 1940
     (1977).
20. R.T.C. Oliver, The Place of Chemotherapy in the Treatment of
     Patients with Invasive Carcinoma of the Bladder, in "Bladder
     Tumors and Other Topics in Urological Oncology", M. Pavone-
     Macaluso, P.H. Smith, F. Edsmyr, eds. Plenum Press, New York,
     pp 381-385 (1980).
21. M. Pavone-Macaluso and EORTC Genitourinary Tract Cooperative
     Group A, Single Drug Chemotherapy of Bladder Cancer with Adria-
     mycin, VM-26, or Bleomycin. A Phase II Multicentric Cooperative
     Study, Eur. Urol. 2: 138 (1976).
22. L.H. Rodriguez, D.E. Johnson, P.Y. Holoye et al, Combination
     VM-26 and Adriamycin for Metastatic Transitional Cell Carcinoma,
     Cancer Treat. Rep. 61: 87 (1977).
23. S. Sakamoto, J. Ogata, K. Ikegami et al, Chemotherapy for Bladder
     Cancer with Neocarcinostatin, Eur. J. Cancer 22: 103 (1980).
24. M.L. Samuels, CISCA Combination Chemotherapy in "2nd Annual
     Conference on Cancer of the Genitourinary Tract", D.E. Johnson,
     M.L. Samuels, eds., Raven Press, New York, pp 97-106 (1979).
25. M.L. Samuels, C. Logothetis, A. Trindade et al, Cytoxan, Adria-
     mycin and Cisplatinum (CISCA) in Metastatic Bladder Cancer,
     Proc. Amer. Assoc. Cancer Res. 21: 137 (1980).
26. J.A. Smith and W.F. Whitmore, Regional Lymph Node Metastasis
     from Bladder Cancer, J. Urol. (in press).
27. M.S. Soloway, Cis-diamminedichloroplatinum (II) (DDP) in
     Advanced Bladder Cancer, J. Urol. 120: 716 (1978).
28. M.S. Soloway and W.M. Murphy, Experimental Chemotherapy of
     Bladder Cancer - Systemic and Intravesical, Sem. Oncol. 6: 168
     (1979).
29. J.J. Sternberg, R.B. Bracken, P.B. Handel et al, Combination
     Chemotherapy (CISCA) for Advanced Urinary Tract Carcinoma. A
     Preliminary Report, JAMA 238: 2282 (1977)
30. A.G. Turner, W.F. Hendry, G.B. Williams et al, The Treatment of
     Advanced Bladder Cancer with Methotrexate, Brit. J. Urol. 49:
     673 (1977).
31. S.D. Williams, L.H. Einhorn, J.P. Donohue, Cis-platinum Combina-
     tion Chemotherapy of Bladder Cancer, Cancer Clin. Trials,
     Cancer Chemotherapy 2: 355 (1979).
32. A. Yagoda, Future Implications of Phase II Chemotherapy Trials
     in ninety-five Patients with Measurable Advanced Bladder Cancer,
     Cancer Res. 37: 2275 (1977).
33. A. Yagoda, R.C. Watson, H. Grabstald, W.E. Barzell and W.F.
     Whitmore, Adriamycin and Cyclophosphamide in Advanced Bladder
     Cancer, Cancer Treat. Rep. 61: 31 (1977b).

34. A. Yagoda, Chemotherapy of Metastatic Bladder Cancer, <u>Cancer</u>
     45: 1879 (1980).
35. A. Yagoda, R.C. Watson, Gonzalez-Vitale et al, Cis-dichloro-
     diammineplatinum (II) in Advanced Bladder Cancer, <u>Cancer Treat.</u>
     <u>Rep</u>. 60: 917 (1976).
36. A. Yagoda, R.C. Watson, W.F. Whitmore et al, Adriamycin in
     Advanced Urinary Tract Cancer, <u>Cancer</u> 39: 279 (1977a).
37. A. Yagoda, R.C. Watson, N. Kemeny et al, Diamminedichloride
     Platinum II and Cyclophosphamide in the Treatment of Advanced
     Urothelial Cancer, <u>Cancer</u> 41: 2121 (1978).
38. A. Yagoda, R.C. Watson, W.F. Whitmore, Phase II Trial of
     Methotrexate in Urinary Bladder Cancer, <u>Proc. Amer. Assoc.</u>
     <u>Cancer Res</u>. 21: 427 (1980a).
39. A. Yagoda, R.C. Watson, R. Blumenreich et al, Phase II Trials
     in Urothelial Tumors with AMSA and PALA, <u>Proc. Amer. Assoc.</u>
     <u>Cancer Res</u>. 21: 427 (1980b).

IMMUNOLOGY

CHAIRMAN'S SUMMARY

J A MARTINEZ-PIÑEIRO

Profesor Agregado, Servicio de Urologia, C.S. La Paz,
Facultad de Medicina, Universidad Autonoma, Madrid,
Spain

Clinical and experimental evidence have repeatedly demonstrated
the relationship between the immune system and the natural history
of cancer; however, it will still be a long time before the intri-
cacies of this relationship are well understood.

The type, number and structure of the cancer cell surface
antigens, against which the immune system is supposed to react, are
poorly known. In the particular case of bladder cancer, a specific
cell surface-bound antigenicity has been demonstrated, implying the
existence of "strange" antigens, as well as the lack of normal A, B,
O, and H antigens on the surface of tumors of high aggressiveness.
There seems also to be evidence suggesting that cancer cell-surface
antigens can, in the course of time, change from high to low antigenicity, as part of the tumor escape mechanism aimed at deceiving
the immune system and thus facilitating its own growth.

The exact nature of the immunologic reaction also remains
obscure. Monocytes (macrophages), and T and B Lymphocytes are
considered to be the basic elements of both the cell-mediated and
the antibody-mediated (humoral) immune response, which comprises
anti-tumor as well as tumor growth enhancing responses; from the
balance of modulation of both will depend the future of the tumor
and, certainly, of the host. The factors modulating the activity
of the helper and suppressor cells, of cytotoxic antibodies, and of
other soluble principles, such as lymphokines and cytotoxicity-
blocking-complexes, are presently unknown. It is likely that gen-
etic factors, linked to the HLA system of incompatibility, will
play a role in this modulation. The familial tendency to cancer
and the association of demonstrable HLA alterations in some types of
human cancers seem to uphold this view.

A depression of the immune response, correlated to the stage
of the disease, has been firmly established but, again, its exact
significance is not well understood. Future clinical longitudinal
studies of the immunologic profile may shed some light on this
problem, if and when the present lack of appropriate monitors to
establish such profiles can be overcome. In effect, skin tests,
either with sensitizing haptenes like DNCB or with recall antigens
and inflammatory agents, are simple and universally used tests, but
are non-specific and too rough to permit the assessment of small
modifications of the cell-mediated immune response; on the other
hand, the more precise and reliable in-vitro tests, designed to
evaluate specifically both the cell - and humoral-mediated responses,
are complex assays, within the reach only of selected investigative
groups and not devoid of imperfections. Clinicians have presently
to rely upon skin tests and a few in-vitro tests, such as the T and
B rosette, the lymphocyte blastogenic stimulation, and the leukocyte
migration inhibition assays.

Poor as it currently is, the assessment of the immune response
is nonetheless relevant for a better knowledge of the natural history
of both untreated and of treated cancers; cancer progression and
cancer therapy (be it surgery, radiotherapy or chemotherapy and
even immunotherapy) are by themselves immuno-depressants and afford
a rationale to try to improve the immunologic defensive capacity by
therapeutic means.

Immunotherapy offers a new approach in cancer therapy, because
it is not directed against the tumor, as are all other therapies,
but towards improving the immune response of the host to help him
fight the tumor. Unfortunately for the present bladder cancer suf-
ferers, immunotherapy is in its infancy: specific stimulation of the
immune system (be it active or passive) is still in the experimental
phase, and non-specific stimulation with chemical agents, vaccines
and bacterial products, although encouraging, has yet to prove its
value in controlled clinical trials. Intravesical BCG therapy for
the prevention of papillary tumor recurrences seems to deserve such
a trial.

In advising groups considering future trials, one thing has to
be kept in mind about immunotherapy: the immune system is only cap-
able of coping with around 10^6 cancer cells. This means that immuno-
stimulation has sense only when it is aimed, as Mathé has pointed
out, at killing the "last cell".

HOST EVALUATION OF PATIENTS WITH BLADDER CANCER

A T LACHAND AND J AUVERT

Service Urologie Mondart
Creteil (Paris)
France

SUMMARY

Evaluation of the general resistance of the patient at the time
of diagnosis, and before proposing treatment and giving a prognosis,
is a very old established medical practice. For two millenia this
host evaluation was based on two notions. One was objective - the
age of the patient, and the other more subjective - the general
appearance of the patient which the physician learned to evaluate from
experience. With the recent growth of Immunology we are beginning to
understand the complex phenomena which inhibit the development of
malignant clones in all animals. The study of the immune defences
adds a third element to this host evaluation.

HOST VERSUS TUMOR DEFENCES

It is more than likely that the organism is permanently and
naturally protecting itself against the development of malignancy.
We know that a lot of malignant cells are circulating in the blood
stream of every cancer bearer but that most will be destroyed before
initiating any metastases. Examples of spontaneous regression of
malignant tumors (32) are also confirming the existence of these
defence mechanisms.

Defence Factors

Some defence factors are not immunological and they are very
well known, including the "physiological" rather than "chronological"
age. The age of the patient is very important in the choice of a
treatment since major surgery, e.g. total cystectomy, will be avoided
in those with only a short life expectancy. The relationship between

127

the age of the patients and spontaneous resistance to malignancy
remains unclear; indeed some malignant tumors seem to grow faster in
young people. The nutritional state of the patients is another
important factor. The better it is, the better will the patient
resist the development of the tumor and its possible infectious
complications (9, 36).

These factors, which reflect the general status of the patients,
are also influencing his immune defences. The weakening of these
defences associated with increasing age is a classical concept (5,65)
but although some studies confirm this idea (55) not all authors
accept it (12). The relationship between nutritional state, plasma
albumin level, total protein mass and immune status have recently
been extensively studied (9,16,36,58,89).

Immunity

The role of immunity is well established. Its importance can
be judged from:-

(a) The well known suppression of cutaneous delayed hypersensitivity
reactions, in Hodgkin disease and in several other reticulo-endothelial malignancies.

(b) The greater frequency of malignant tumors in naturally or
pharmacologically immuno-depressed patients (14,62). In this
situation leukemias or hematosarcomas are often seen but other solid
tumors may also be observed (26).

(c) The transfer of anti-tumoral immunity by injection of immune
lymphocytes rather than specific antibodies in laboratory animals
(60). Following this idea some authors (84) have treated advanced
bladder tumors by intra-arterial injection of pig lymphocytes
previously sensitized to these same tumors. Such a treatment appears
to us to be very hazardous but it is impossible to deny that a
permanent anti-tumor immunological surveillance does exist in normal
subjects.

General Anti-tumor Immunity

Fig. 1 shows the principal mechanisms of anti-tumor immunity.
Tumor antigens are recognised by the macrophages or by the T-lymphocytes and T-lymphocytes are stimulated by this recognition. They
multiply (cell-immunity) and they help B-lymphocytes in antibody
synthesis. Stimulated T-lymphocytes may exert their cytotoxic
power either directly or through macrophages. For this purpose they
secrete lymphokines which help macrophages to stay close to the tumor
cells and a "macrophage arming factor" which make them cytotoxic.
These mechanisms represent the essential part of immune surveillance
(24,31).

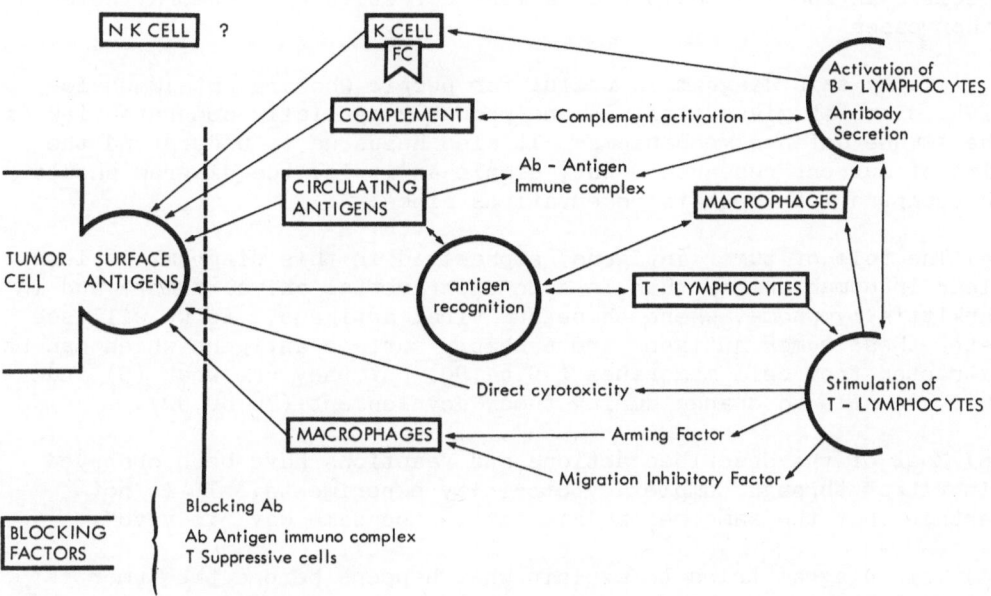

Fig. 1.   The principal mechanisms of anti-tumor immunity.

However, the role of humoral immunity also seems to be important.
Antibodies intervene in T-lymphocyte and macrophage activation.
Combining with tumor-cell surface antigens they lead to cell
destruction through the activation of complement (41) or by means of
K-cells (88). Droller (24) wrote recently on a possible role of
interferon which would enhance the cytotoxic action of K-cells and
T-lymphocytes.

The existence of immune complex blocking cytotoxicity reactions
and helping tumor growth seems to be experimentally proven (1,45).
On the other hand neutralisation of circulating tumor antigens by
specific antibodies could play a more effective anti-tumoral role in
other cases (45).

Today this diagram is useful for people who are not immunolo-
gists since it gives a simple and probably partially accurate view of
the immune defence mechanisms. It also helps us to understand the
aims of current research. But, simple as it is, the diagram should
be accepted with certain reservations since:-

(a) The role of tumor antigens, emphasized in this diagram, is less
clear in human tumors than in some experimental animal tumors and in
Burkitt's lymphoma, where these are viral antigens. As we will see
later these tumor antigens are probably surface antigens which can be
extracted from cell membranes (19,64,90) but they are weak (5) and
they are able to change during tumor development (70,80,92).

(b) Most of the described actions and reactions have been observed
"in vitro" through complex cytotoxicity experiments. It is not
certain that the same mechanisms act in the same way "in vivo".

(c) This diagram tries to explain what happens before the tumor is
organised, i.e. when there are still very few abnormal cells. But in
human medicine we are facing patients bearing macroscopic tumors
which have already broken through the first immune defences. This
situation is probably quite different. It is also likely that a
tumor, as it becomes bigger, secretes some factors able to enhance
its own growth and which are different from immune complexes. The
role of circulating peptides is suggested by the work of Glasgow (37)
and of Constantian (20). The action of T-suppressive cells (5,53)
would also preserve tumor growth and finally the reduction in levels
of some alpha-2 glyco proteins which are induced by tumor growth or
by surgical operations could also modify immune defences (77).

Inflammatory phenomena in anti-tumoral defences

The potential importance of such phenomena is suggested by the
infiltration of some tumors with polynuclear cells but their role is
not well understood. The level of inflammatory response can be
studied by skin sensitization tests using croton oil. They are

thought not to be correlated with the skin tests of immunity (51). Brosman et al (12) used these tests in patients with bladder tumors but did not obtain any clear cut results. The sedimentation rate is also of some interest, especially for the follow up of papillary tumors, but it is not very specific.

With the kind help of Professor Boigne, we used an immuno-nephelemetric method to measure the serum concentrations of Haptglobin and alpha-1 antitrypsin in 61 patients with different genito-urinary malignancies. (Fig. 2). The serum levels of these two proteins are generally considered as reflecting the inflammatory response. The levels were elevated in 48 patients and normal in 13 patients. These 13 patients had small tumors with no metastases. Of the 48 patients whose levels were elevated, 37 had large or widespread tumors. These proteins were measured in 28 bladder tumor patients of whom 9 had normal levels; all nine patients had non-invasive papillary tumors. The 19 patients with elevated levels of the relevant proteins all had invasive or disseminated tumors. We believe that the serum levels of haptoglobin and of alpha 1 - antitrypsin are too directly correlated with tumor extent to have a real prognostic value. However the relationship between inflammatory response and tumor growth is certainly worthy of more extensive study.

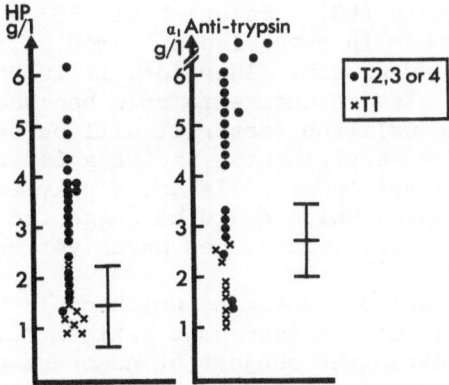

Fig. 2.   Serum inflammatory proteins - 27 patients with transitional
          cell tumors.

IMMUNOLOGICAL PATTERNS IN PATIENTS WITH TRANSITIONAL CELL CARCINOMA

Since 1970 the immune reactions of bladder carcinomas have been extensively studied.

Antigens related to bladder tumor cells

Initially Bubenik (13) proved the existence of specific antigens on papillary tumors. Following Rigby's research (74) he began "in vitro" culture of a cell-line originating in a human bladder cancer. Ten years later this cell-line is still living following successive sub-cultures and the cultivated cells are still believed to carry the same antigens. During these ten years several other research teams have used cells from Bubenik's cell-line (6,42,88) and additional cell-lines, originating in other bladder cancers, have been established "in vitro". In December 1978 Fogh (34) and Elliott (29) reported on 23 bladder cancer cell-lines.

The antigens are probably mainly surface antigens as suggested by Johansson (50) who showed immunoglobulins bound to the cell surface in some bladder tumors and by Pizza (70) who stated that tumoral cells, when preserved for months in formal-dehyde at 4°, kept their antigenicity unchanged. DcCenzo et al (22) showed A, B and H antigens on the surface of normal transitional cells (94). Disappearance of these normal surface antigens in papillary tumors indicates a poor prognosis. This work was confirmed by other authors (2,10,57,71,73, 78,94,95) and has great practical interest as it represents a new prognostic factor. From a theoretical point of view it is likely that, in tumors with a bad prognosis, the A, B and H antigens are replaced by abnormal tumor antigens.

Nuclear abnormalities, which are found more frequently in the aggressive tumors (59) might act as other tumor antigens, but it is felt that this is unlikely (60). Falor et al (33) have isolated a specific chromosome marker in some bladder tumor cells, the presence of which implies a bad prognosis. Therefore it is unlikely that this chromosome marker will play an antigenic role because the richer the antigenicity of a tumor cell the faster it will be detected and destroyed. We know of no experimental fact suggesting that any abnormalities of DNA or RNA tumor cells could play an antigenic role. The role of viruses, which could be suggested by the evolutional pattern of papillary tumors, has never yet been demonstrated.

Among circulating soluble antigens which could be secreted by bladder tumors only one, Carcinoembryonic antigen (C.E.A.) has been frequently detected and was the subject of numerous papers (35,38,43, 49,93). Increased levels were found more often in the urine than in the serum, ranging from 25 - 80% of patients according to different authors. Measurement of C.E.A. would perhaps be useful in the follow up of patients after transurethral resection of papillary tumor.

Recently Guinan et al (40) stated that the plasma level of C.E.A. is higher than 2.4 nanog./ml in 60% of bladder tumor patients, and the urinary level higher than 9.9 nanog./ml in 36%. However they think that it is not a very specific test because a high urinary level of C.E.A. can be observed even in simple urinary infection.

Therefore, in papillary tumors, it is probably the surface antigens bound to the cell membranes which play the first role in initiating the immune response (48). However for a given tumor it is likely that the antigens can change with time and that the antigenic power of the first tumor is greater than that of subsequent recurrences, as suggested by Pizza (70). On the other hand, antigenic power remains unchanged in the "in vitro" cultured cell-line. Therefore it is likely that human tumors enhance their own agressiveness by selecting the less antigenic cell-lines (5,23,70).

Cellular immunity of transitional cell carcinomas

(a) Pathological basis. The importance of cellular immune factors in the defence mechanisms against bladder tumors has for a long time been suggested by the prognostic value of tumor infiltration by round cells (52,79,86). More recently Herr (47) observed that the pathological appearance of the lymph nodes which drain the tumor is of great prognostic interest. The risk of metastases is lower and the chances of five year survival higher if these lymph nodes look "stimulated". Lymph nodes which have a big germinal center and a thick paracortical area, are considered as stimulated. These features suggest an important multiplication of B and T-lymphocytes. However patients whose lymph nodes look depleted or at rest have a higher risk of metastases and a lower life expectancy. This work appears to be of great potential value and it would be desirable for the results to be confirmed by other teams. It is noteworthy that Catalona (17) extracted, from these same lymph nodes, a substance which inhibits the cytotoxicity of K-cells.

(b) Depression of non specific cellular immunity in patients with bladder tumors. Apart from the above mentioned anatomical studies, research on cellular immunity in patients with bladder tumors in the last 10 years has been directed in two main ways - towards non specific immune depression which would enhance tumor growth and towards specific hypersensitivity to tumor antigens which would restrain tumor development.

Depression of immunity may be measured by the total lymphocyte count which is lowered in some cases (3). However this is not very significant (55). It may also be measured by the number of T-lymphocytes using the E. rosette test. the T-lymphocytes may be lowered in patients with bladder tumor, but only in those with widespread disease (1,12).

The patient's lymphocytes may be stimulated by phytohaemag-
glutinin (PHA) or concavallin A (COA) (8). Any reduction in the
blastic transformation can be evaluated optically (75) or by incorp-
oration of H3-Thymidine (63).

Non-specific cytotoxicity has been measured by Brosman and
Ehlilali (12,28) who studied in vitro cytotoxicity of patients'
lymphocytes in mice. Their results were inconclusive.

Other in vitro tests (including graft versus host reactions
(82), study of chemotaxis of monocytes (44), and measurement of
adenosine-deaminase activity of lymphocytes (83) have been used to
confirm the weakening of immune defences.

The most extensively studied are the in vivo skin tests of
delayed hypersensitivity. They can be divided into two groups:-

(i) intra-dermal injection of common antigens that the patient has
probably already met - recall antigens (tuberculin, extracts of
dermatophytes, candida, streptococcus, mumps) which study the immune
memory and
(ii) skin tests using DNCB which require previous sensitization
because it is an antigen that the patient has usually not previously
met. As a result, two stages are necessary. In the first, sensitization is produced by application of 2000 μg of DNCNB to the skin.
In the second, 14 days later, the skin is tested by application of 25
or 100 μg. The strength of this skin reaction will evaluate the
organisms' ability to immunise itself against new antigens (18).

These skin tests are safe and easy to do. They were studied in
large series of patients with bladder carcinoma as well as in
patients with other kinds of tumors (8,12,16,67,80). All these
studies showed a higher incidence of anergic subjects among patients
than in a control group. A correlation between the stage of the
tumor and the incidence of non-reactivity should exist. In addition,
these studies suggest that these skin tests may perhaps be of value
in prognosis.

Skin tests using DNCB sensitisation are time consuming, more
complex than those using simple recall antigens and are sometimes
responsible for allergic accidents but they appear to be more
reliable (8,12,27), as less than 10% of people in a control population are DNCB negative. On the other hand, tests using recall
antigens are more simple and are always safe in spite of the fact
that they are "in vivo" tests. They are also reliable if each intra-
dermal test is read, not in isolation, but collectively as part of a
battery of three or more skin tests (50,54,55,56,36). In this way
the incidence of anergic subjects in control groups is lower than 20%
(55).

We studied secondary cell immunity using skin tests with three recall antigens 70 times in 57 patients with bladder tumors. We used the following simple protocol. An intra-dermal injection of 10 units of tuberculin (PPD) is read 48 and 72 hours later. If induration or erythema is larger than 5 mm the skin test is considered positive and the patient non anergic. Nothing more needs to be done. If the reaction is smaller, two further intradermal injections are then given - of candidine 10^{-4} (0.1 ml) and varidase (100 units of streptokinase and 25 units of streptodornase in 0.1 ml) and read 48 hours later.

The patient is said to be anergic only if the sum of the three intradermal reactions does not reach 5 mm.

In this study the mean age of the 57 patients was 65 years. Fourteen patients had T1 papillary tumors and 43 patients had invasive tumors. Among these 16 had lymph node invasion or metastases. Only 8 patients were anergic and 2 more became secondarily anergic. This incidence, when compared to that found in other tumors, seems to be low and transitional cell carcinoma does not appear to affect the skin test responses as much as other malignancies, e.g. prostatic cancer (54) (Table 1). Furthermore, all the anergic patients had large invasive tumors with the exception of one patient over 80 years of age with a category T3 lesion. The clear correlation of the results of these skin tests with tumor stage greatly diminish their prognostic value. Nevertheless when we isolate the 39 patients with invasive carcinomas to whom active treatment was given, we see that the mortality rate in this group was higher in anergic patients. But it is too small a group to yield a definite conclusion. However, when we compare the actuarial survival lines of the anergic and non-anergic patients (after exclusion of a T1 non invasive tumor) there appears a statistically significant difference (Fig. 3).

Table 1
Prognostic value of skin tests on 39 patients with invasive carcinoma in whom active treatment (surgery or radiotherapy) was undertaken.

Tests	Died within 3 months	Died within 12 months
0	5/7	6/6
+	4/32	16/25

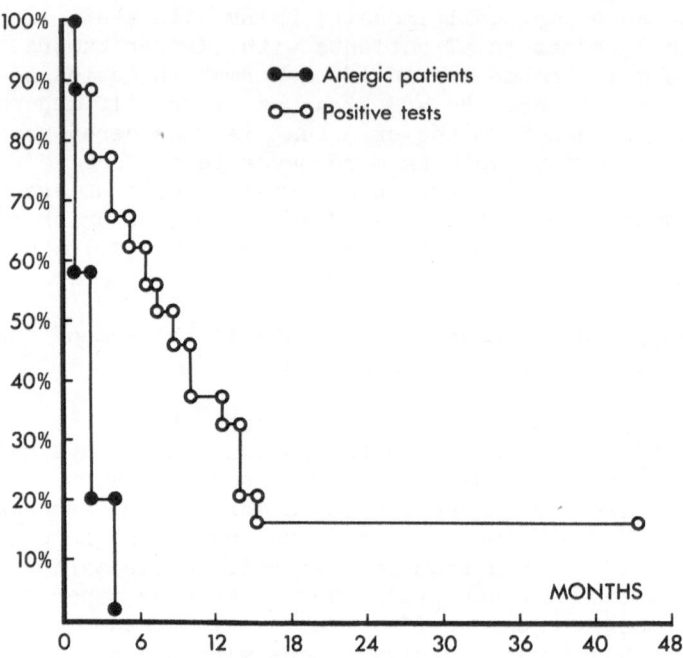

Fig. 3.   Actuarial survival of 43 patients with invasive bladder
cancer according to Immunological Status.

In conclusion, skin tests with recall antigen are not useful in
patients with non invasive papillary tumors, because these tumors do
not cause any immune depression detectable by this method. Invasive
transitional cell carcinomas lead to immune depression less
frequently or later than in other uro-genital malignancies,
especially prostatic cancer. However if immune depression is seen,
it is of ominous prognostic significance.

(c) Specific cell immunity against tumor antigens. Several authors
have shown that circulating lymphocytes of patients with bladder
tumors have a greater in vitro cytotoxic activity against allogeneic
bladder tumor cultivated cells (13,68,91) and that the increased
cytotoxicity is specific: patients' lymphocytes are aggressive
against a cell line whose origin is in a bladder cancer, but show
normal reactivity against other target cells.

This toxicity can be studied in vitro in two ways - by observing the growth inhibition of target cells through a microscope (5,42,85, 91) or by measuring the radio activity of supernatant liquid over cultured cells previously labelled with Cr 51, H3 - proline or H3-Thymidine (5,8,12,46,88). The concordance of results obtained by different teams gives a great interest to these cytotoxicity experiments. Furthermore some groups made an attempt to show that cytotoxicity would vary with the stage of the disease - very strong in superficial tumors and weak in invasive tumors (7,46,66,68). This leads us to hope that these cytotoxicity tests will perhaps have a prognostic value in the future. However, these experiments are difficult, expensive and time consuming. Their reproducibility is uncertain and depends on target-cell quality (6,12,29,34,66,91). They can only be carried out in laboratories equipped for immunological research and consequently are not routinely performed and are still not able to give us reliable information. Furthermore, it is amazing to learn that there is no good agreement between these in vitro tests and skin tests (80).

Stimulation of patients' lymphocytes by tumor cells in "in vitro" mixed culture was studied by Cummings (21) and Pizza (70) and showed a greater stimulation if specific antigens were present on the stimulating cells. Inhibition of migration of the patient's leukocytes either by cultivation of tumor cells (70) or by their membrane extracts (81) confirms the importance and the specificity of surface antigens. In addition, inhibition of leukocyte adherence by tumor antigens has been studied by Vetto (90) and by Guinan (39).

Humoral Immunity in Transitional Cell Carcinoma

Measurement of the serum concentrations of immunoglobulins and of some fractions of the complement system has been undertaken by several authors without any conclusive result. With the kind help of Professor Boigne we measured plasma levels of IgG, IgA, IgM and the C3 fraction of the complement in 27 patients with bladder tumors (Fig. 4). Among our results we noted

(a) a slight elevation of IgA concentration in 8/27 patients. All eight had invasive tumors.

(b) a slight elevation of IgM in 6/27 patients and of C3 in 10/27 patients. The majority of these patients had T1 non invasive tumors.

Perhaps these recent results suggest a slight elevation of humoral immune defences in the early stages of the disease. However it is obvious that the differences are too little and our series too short to allow us to draw definitive conclusions.

Circulating antibodies were found by some authors (30,61) but not by others (69). Hakala et al (42) found an antibody in patients' serum which was able to enhance lymphocyte cytotoxicity in other

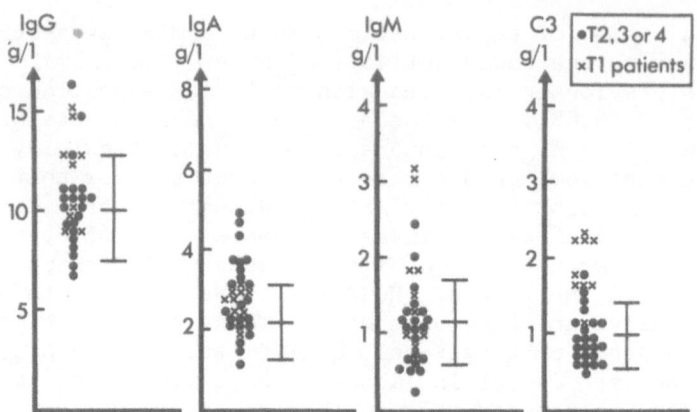

Fig. 4. Immunoglobulins and C3 fraction of the complement in the
         serum of 27 patients with bladder tumors.

patients bearing the same kind of tumor. This finding awaits
confirmation.

     It is now clear that the most important part of the in vitro
lymphocyte cytotoxicity against allogeneic target cells is due to K-
cells wearing Fc receptors, and that an antibody is necessary to let
these K-cells exert their cytotoxic role (46,88) (antibody dependent
cytotoxicity). These "in vitro" results may probably be transposed
"in vivo" in spite of the fact that "in vivo" macrophages, T-lymphocytes and complement are probably active in addition to the K-cells.
Consequently, <u>cytotoxicity</u> which appears to be the most important
part of the anti-tumoral cell immunity system <u>depends on a circulating antibody</u>.

     Droller (24) recently showed that human interferon would
enhance direct and antibody dependent cytotoxicity. Also McLaughlin
(63), working on lymphocyte stimulation by phyto hemagglutinin,
showed that some patients with bladder tumors have low values and
that it is possible to transfer this depression to lymphocytes of
normal people by means of a plasma exchange. Consequently, a factor
inhibiting lymphocyte reactivity must exist in the plasma, almost
certainly an α2 globulin. There seems to be no doubt that cell
immunity and humoral immunity both play important roles in the host
defences against bladder tumors.

CONCLUSIONS

     During the last ten years bladder tumors have been extensively
studied from an immunological point of view. From this extensive
research two ideas have emerged:-

1. Bladder tumor cells carry surface antigens which are fairly specific. It is possible that these antigens lead to a specific immune response at the beginning of the disease.

2. Patients with widespread invasive bladder cancer show a reduction in the total non specific immune defences, as commonly seen in solid tumors. This immune depression is neither earlier nor more extensive in transitional cell carcinoma than in other tumors.

These two ideas have a great theoretical interest and we may hope that further progress in tumor immunology will eventually bring us an early method for the detection of recurrences, or even a preventive treatment through a kind of vaccination. However it is still too early to draw any firm conclusions.

Non specific immune stimulation, using bacterial antigens, Levamisole or other products although safe is not yet of proven efficacy. In patients who are to undergo a major surgical operation and who are anergic it would be interesting to study the effects of pre operative immune stimulation, because it seems clear that anergy enhances the risk of surgical and infective complications (36). However the utlilisation of tumor extracts "in vivo" must be forbidden until we can predict whether such injection will enhance or inhibit the desired immune response which may be affected by immune complexes, blocking antigens, saturation of antibodies, or stimulation of suppressive cells. In tumor immunology a lot of questions still remain unanswered.

Urological groups which are lucky enough to work with laboratories of Immunology must continue the research which has just been briefly summarised and especially that concerned with cytotoxicity experiments. Because bladder tumors are frequent and need repeated resections they are a ready source of cellular material which can be cultured in nude mice, in the cheek pouch of the hamster, or in vitro. Therefore transitional cell carcinoma is a most suitable field for research in tumor immunology.

Urologists who are not associated with such laboratories cannot undertake such in vitro or animal research. However, from the topics which have been mentioned above, we would like to propose to them five subjects for research:-

1. To develop and improve skin tests, using either DNCB or other recall antigens, in patients with invasive bladder cancer and more especially when major surgery is foreseen, in order to detect and to try to correct a possible general immune depression which would have a bad prognostic significance.

2. Measurement of plasma and urinary levels of C.E.A. is now easy and is becoming less expensive. Consequently, determination of this

marker should be encouraged and may perhaps help us to detect early recurrences after tumor ablation.

3. To continue the study of the inflammatory reaction and its relationship with immune defences, by means of systematic measurement of the parameters of inflammation such as sedimentation rate, croton oil skin tests, Haptoglobin, alpha-1-antitrypsin, alpha-2-macroglobulin and fibrin.

4. To develop the study of A, B and H antigens in papillary tumors. Their detection technique is now accurate. These antigens, besides their great theoretical interest in tumor antigenicity, seem to have a real prognostic value.

5. If a cystectomy is performed, ask for a very accurate lymph node study, not only to search for metastases but also to know whether or not the nodes are "stimulated", in order to confirm the work of Herr (47) and to obtain a new element in prognosis.

      None of these five suggestions contains any risk for our patients. The cost is low and they may be carried out by any urological team. Therefore, we think that these propositions should be considered. They could probably bring to Urologists a better understanding of the host-versus-tumor mechanisms and a better evaluation of tumoral and therapeutic risk for each of our patients.

REFERENCES

1.   H. Akaza, H. Yokoyama, T. Umeda and T. Nijima, Restoration by Levamizole of E Rosette Formation and its Abrogation by Autochtonous Serum from Patients with Bladder Cancer, Cancer, 43: 97 (1979).
2.   J. Alroy, K. Teramura, A.W. Miller, B.V. Pauli et al, Isoantigens A, B and H in Urinary Bladder Carcinoma Following Radiotherapy, Cancer 41: 1739 (1978).
3.   M. Amin and R. Lich, Lymphocytes and Bladder Cancer, J. Urol, 111: 165 (1974).
4.   F.H. Bach, Normal Histocompatibility Antigens as a Model for Tumors, Am. J. Clin. Path. 62: 173 (1974).
5.   J.F. Bach, Immunologie, Vol. 1, Flammarion Médecine-Sciences, Paris (1976).
6.   M.A. Bean, R.B. Bloom, R.B. Herberman, L.J. Old et al, Cell-mediated Cytotoxicity for Bladder Carcinoma: Evaluation of a Workshop, Cancer Res. 35: 2902 (1975).
7.   M.A. Bean, H. Pees, J.E. Fogh, H. Grabstald and H.F. Oeetgen, Cytotoxicity of Lymphocytes from Patients with Cancer of the Bladder. Detection by a 3H-Prolene Microcytotoxicity Test, Int. J. Cancer, 14: 186 (1974).

8. M.A. Bean, P.S. Schellhammer, H.W. Herr, C.M. Pinsky and W.K. Whitmore, Immunocompetence of Patients with Transitional Cell Carcinomas as Measured by DNCB Skin Tests and In Vitro Lymphocytes Functions, Nat. Cancer Inst. Monographs, 49: 111 (1978).

9. J. Belghiti, G. Champault, F. Fabre and J.C. Patel, Appréciation du Risque Infectieux Post-opératoire par les Tests D'Hypersensibilité Retardée, N. Presse Med. 7: 3337 (1978).

10. S. Bergman and N. Javadpour, The Cell Surface Antigens A, B or O(H) as an Indicator of Malignant Potential in Stage A Bladder Carcinoma: Preliminary Report, J. Urol. 119: 49 (1978).

11. B.R. Bistrian, M. Sherman, G.L. Blackburn, R. Marshall and C. Shaw, Cellular Immunity in Adult Marasmus, Arch. Intern. Med. 137: 1408 (1977).

12. S. Brosman, M. Elhilali, C. Vescera and J. Fahey, Immune Response in Bladder Cancer Patients, J. Urol. 121: 162 (1979).

13. J. Bubenik, P. Perlmann, K. Helmstein and G. Moberger, Immune Response to Urinary Bladder Tumours in Men, Int. J. Cancer, 5: 39 (1970).

14. M. Burnet, Immunological Factors in the Process of Carcinogenesis, Brit. Med. Bull. 20: 154 (1964).

15. F.B. Burt, M. Pavone-Macaluso, J.W. Horns and J.J. Kaufman, Heterotransplantation of Bladder Cancer in the Hamster Cheek Pouch: In Vivo Testing of Cancer Chemotherapeutic Agents, J. Urol. 95: 51 (1966).

16. W.J. Catalona and P.B. Chretien, Correlation Among Host Immunocompetence and Tumor Stage, Tumor Grade and Vascular Permeation in Transitional Carcinoma, J. Urol. 110: 526 (1973).

17. W.J. Catalona and A. Feldman, Effect of Regional Node Suppressor Factors on Antibody Dependent Cellular Toxicity, Presented at the 72nd Annual Meeting of the A.U.A. - Chicago,April (1977).

18. W.J. Catalona, P.T. Taylor, A.S. Rabson and P.B. Chretein, A Method for Dinitrochlorobenzene Contact Sensitization: A Clinicopath. Study, New Engl. J. Med. 286: 399 (1972).

19. D.H. Char, A. Hollinshead and R.B. Herberman, Skin Tests with Soluble Antigens in Patients with Choroidal Tumors, Cancer 40: 1650 (1977).

20. M.B. Constantian, Association of Sepsis with an Immunosuppressive Polypeptide in the Serum of Burn Patients, Ann. Surg. 188: 209 (1978).

21. K.B. Cummings, Y. Kodera and M.A. Bean, In Vitro Immune Parameters in Relation to Clinical Course in Transitional Cells Carcinomas, Nat. Cancer Instit. Monographs, 49: 119 (1978).

22. J.M. Decenzo and G.W. Leadbetter, The Interaction of Host Immunocompetence and Tumor Aggressiveness in Superficial Bladder Carcinoma, J. Urol. 115: 262 (1976).

23. J.B. DeKernion, The Status of Tumor Immunotherapy in Genitourinary Cancer, in "Genitourinary cancer", Skinner and DeKernion eds., W.B. Saunders Co., Philadelphia (1978).

24. M.J. Droller, H. Borg and P. Perlmann, In Vitro Enhancement of Natural and Antibody Dependent Lymphocyte-mediated Cytotoxicity Against Tumor Target Cells by Interferon, Cell. Immunol. 47: 248 (1979).

25. M.J. Droller and J.S. Remington, A Role for the Macrophages in In Vivo and In Vitro Resistance to Murine Bladder Tumor Cell Growth, Cancer Res. 35: 49 (1975).

26. F.R. Eilber and D.L. Morton, Impaired Immunologic Reactivity and Recurrence Following Cancer Surgery, Cancer, 25: 362 (1970).

27. F.R. Eilber, J.A. Nizze and D.L. Morton, Sequential Evaluation of General Immune Competence in Cancer Patients: Correlation with Clinical Course, Cancer, 35: 660 (1975).

28. M.M. Elhilali, S. Britton, S. Brosman and J.F. Fahey, Critical Evaluation of Lymphocyte Functions in Urological Cancer Patients Cancer Res. 36: 132 (1976).

29. A.Y. Elliott, D.L. Bronson and E.E. Fraley, Nat. Cancer Inst. Monographs, 49: 23 (1978)

30. A.Y. Elliott, S. Dombrovski and E.E. Fraley, Transitional Cell Carcinoma: Fluorescent Antibody Binding to Tumor Cells, Nat. Cancer Inst. Monographs, 49: 199 (1978).

31. R. Evans and P. Alexander, Mechanism of Immunologically Specific Killing of Tumor Cells by Macrophages, Nature, 236: 168 (1972).

32. T.C. Everson and W.H. Cole, Spontaneous Regression of Cancer, W.B. Saunders Co., Philadelphia (1966)

33. W.H. Falor and R.M. Ward, Prognosis in Early Carcinoma of the Bladder Based on Chromosomal Analysis, J. Urol. 119: 44 (1978).

34. J. Fogh, Cultivation, Characterisation and Identification of Human Tumor Cells, Nat. Cancer Inst. Monographs, 49: 5 (1978).

35. R.A. Fraser, M.J. Ravry, J.W. Segura and V.L.W. Go, Clinical Evaluation of Urinary and Serum Carcinoembryonnic Antigen in Bladder Cancer, J. Urol. 114: 226 (1975).

36. C. George, Intérêt des Tests Cutanés Explorant L'Immunité Cellulaire chez les Malades Hospitalisés en Réanimation et en Chirurgie, Concours Medical, 102: 1181 (1980).

37. A.H. Glasgow, R.B. Nimberg, J.O. Menzoian, Z.I. Saporoschetz et al, Association of Energy with an Immunosuppressive Peptide Fraction in the Serum of Patients with Cancer, New. Engl. J. Med. 291: 1263 (1974).

38. P. Guinan, T. John, N. Sadoughi, R.J. Ablin and I. Bush, Urinary Carcinoembryonnic like Antigen Levels in Patients with Bladder Cancer, J. Urol. 111: 350 (1974).

39. P. Guinan, C. McKiel, M. Flanagan, R. Bhatti, D. Pessis and R.J. Ablin, Cellular Immunity in Bladder Cancer Patients, J. Urol. 119: 747 (1978).

40. P. Guinan, C.McKiel, A. Sundar, R. Veith, A. Dubin and R.J. Ablin, The Carcinoembryonnic Antigen Test in Urologic Cancers, Nat. Cancer Inst. Monographs, 49: 225 (1978).

41. T.R. Hakala, A.B. Castro, A.Y. Elliott and E.E. Fraley, Humoral Cytotoxicity in Human Transitional Cell Carcinoma, J. Urol. 111: 382 (1974).

42. T.R. Hakala, P.H. Lange, A.B. Castro, A.Y. Elliott and E.E. Fraley, Antibody Induction of Lymphocyte-mediated Cytotoxicity Against Human Transitional Cell Carcinomas of the Urinary Tract, New Engl. J. Med. 291: 637 (1974).

43. R.R. Hall, D.J.R. Laurence, A. Munro Neville and D.M. Wallace, Carcinoembryonnic Antigen in Urothelial Carcinomas, Brit. J. Urol. 45: 88 (1973).

44. M.S. Hausman and S.A. Brosman, Abnormal Monocyte Function in Bladder Cancer Patients, J. Urol. 115: 537 (1976).

45. I. Hellstrom, H.O. Sjügren and G. Warner, Blocking of Cell Mediated Tumor Immunity by Sera from Patients with Growing Neoplasms, Int. J. Cancer, 7: 226 (1971).

46. W.H. Herr, Immunobiology of Human Bladder Cancer, J. Urol. 115: 147 (1976).

47. W.H. Herr, M.A. Bean and W.F. Whitmore, Prognostic Significance of Regional Lymph Node Histology in Cancer of the Bladder, J. Urol. 115: 264 (1976).

48. A.C. Hollinshead, Skin Tests with Soluble Tumor Membrane Antigens in Patients with Transitional Cell Cancer, Nat. Cancer Inst. Monographs, 49: 255 (1978).

49. G. Ionescu, N.A. Romas, L. Ionescu, S. Bennette et al, Carcinoembryonnic Antigen and Bladder Carcinoma, J. Urol. 115: 46 (1976).

50. B. Johansson and A. Ljungquist, Localisation of Immunoglobulins in Bladder Tumors, Acta Path. Microb. Scand. 82: 559 (1974).

51. M.W. Johnson, H.I. Mailbach and S.E. Salmon, Skin Reactivity in Patients with Cancer; Impaired Delayed Hypersensitivity or Faulty Inflammatory Response? New Engl. J. Med. 284: 1255 (1971).

52. L.W. Jones and C. O'Toole, Lymphocyte Response to Transitional Cell Carcinoma: Peripheral Cytotoxicity and Local Tumor Infiltration, J. Urol. 118: 974.(1977).

53. J.M. Kirkwood and R.K. Gershon, A Role for Suppressor T Cells in Immunological Enhancement of Tumor Growth, Prog. Exp. Tumor Res. 19: 157 (1974).

54. A.T. Lachand, Bilan Immunologique des Cancer de la Prostate, Ann. Urol. 14: 173 (1980).

55. A.T. Lachand and C. Martin-Mondieres, Les Test Cutanés Étudiant L'Immunité Cellulaire Secondaire. Pratique et Intérêt en Carcinologie Urologique, J. Urol. Nephrol. 85: 214 (1979).

56. A.T. Lachand and C. Martin-Mondieres, Immune Evaluation with Skin Tests in Prostatic Carcinomas, Eur. Urol. 5: 117 (1979).

57. P.H. Lange, C. Limas and E.E. Fraley, Tissue Blood-group Antigens and Prognosis in Low Stage Transitional Cell Carcinoma of the Bladder, J. Urol. 119: 52 (1978).

58. D.K. Law, S.J. Dudrick and N.I. Abdou, The Effect of Protein-Calorie Malnutrition on Immune Competence of Surgical Patients, Surg. Gynec. Obstet. 139: 257 (1972).

59. P.E. Levi, E.H. Cooper, C.K. Anderson and R.E. Williams, Analyses of DNA Content, Nuclear Size and Cell Proliferation in TCC in Man, Cancer, 23: 1074 (1969).

60. J.P. Levi, Immunité Antitumorale, in "Immunologie", J.F. Bach ed. Flammarion, Paris (1976).

61. M.G. Lewis and T.M. Phillips, Tumor-specific Antigens in Human Bladder Cancer, Proc. National Bladder Cancer Conference, Miami, 17 (1976).

62. C.F. McKhann, Immunobiology of Cancer, in "Transplantation", J.S. Najarian and R.L. Simmons eds., Lea & Febiger, Philadelphia, p. 297 (1972).

63. A.P. McLaughlin and J.D. Brooks, A Plasma Factor Inhibiting Lymphocytes' Reactivity in Urologic Cancer Patients, J. Urol. 112: 366 (1974).

64. M.S. Meltzer, E.J. Leonard, H.J. Rapp and T. Birsos, Tumor Specific Antigen Solubilisation by Hypertonic Potassium Chloride, J. Nat. Cancer Inst. 47: 730 (1972).

65. R. Moulias and F. Congy, Problèmes Immunologiques du Sujet Agé, Concours Medical, 102: 2223 (1980).

66. P.J. O'Boyle, E.H. Cooper and R.E. Williams, Evaluation of Immunologic Reactivity in Bladder Cancer, Brit. J. Urol. 46: 303 (1974).

67. C.A. Olsson, C.N. Rao, J.O. Menzoian and W.E. Byrd, Immunologic un-reactivity in Bladder Cancer Patients, J. Urol. 107: 607 (1972).

68. C. O'Toole, B. Unsgaard, L.E. Almgard and B. Johansson, The Cellular Immune Response to Carcinoma of the Urinary Bladder. Correlation to Clinical Stage and Therapy, Brit. J. Cancer 28: 266, Suppl. 1 (1973).

69. A.J. Pesce, A. Evans, B.S. Ooi and Y.M. Ooi, Specific Antibodies to Bladder Carcinoma Tumor Antigen, Proc. Nat. Bladder Cancer Conference, Miami, 18 (1976).

70. G. Pizza, D. Viza, M. Fini, D. Cuzzocrea et al, Transitional Cell Carcinoma of the Bladder - Differences Between Primary Tumor and Following Relapses, Eur. Urol. 6: 45 (1980).

71. G. Raymond, Communication to the French Society of Urology - June 1980, in press.

72. G. Reynoso, T.M. Chu, P. Guinan and G.P. Murphy, Carcinoembryonnic Antigen in Patients with Tumors of the Urogenital Tract, Cancer, 30: 1 (1972).

73. J.P. Ritchie, R.D. Blute and J. Waisman, Immunologic Indicators of Prognosis in Bladder Cancer. The Importance of Cell-Surface Antigens, J. Urol. 123: 22 (1980).

74. C.C. Rigby and L.M. Franks, A Human Tissue Culture Cell Line from a Transitional Cell Cancer of Bladder, Brit. J. Cancer, 24: 746 (1970).

75. I. Romics and J. Horvath, Study of Non Specific Lymphocyte Transformation in Urologic Cancer Patients, Int. Urol. Nephrol. 10: 261 (1978).

76. J.A. Roth, F.R. Eilber, J.A. Nizze and D.L. Morton, Lack of Correlation Between Skin Reactivity to D.N.C.B. and Croton Oil in Cancer Patients, New. Engl. J. Med. 293: 388 (1975).

77. T.M. Saba, Prevention of Liver Reticulo-endothelial Systemic
     Host Defence Failure After Surgery by Intravenous Opsonic
     Glyco-protein Therapy, Ann. Surg. 188: 147 (1978).
78. N. Sadoughi, A. Rubenstone, J. Misna and I. Davidsohn, The Cell
     Surface Antigens of Bladder Washing Specimens in Patients with
     Bladder Tumor.   A New Approach, J. Urol. 123: 19 (1980).
79. K.P. Sarma, The Role of Lymphoid Reaction in Bladder Cancer,
     J. Urol. 104: 843 (1970).
80. P.F. Schellhammer, R.B. Bracken, M.A. Bean, C.M. Pinsky and
     W.F. Whitmore, Immune Evaluation with Skin Testing, Cancer,
     38: 149 (1976).
81. P.F. Schellhammer, G.L. Wright, F.E. Rosato and R.J. Faulconer,
     Leucocyte Migration Inhibition Assay in Patients with Bladder
     Carcinoma, J. Urol. 122: 746 (1979).
82. B. Shuhat et al., Cellular Immune Competence in Patients with
     Transitional Cell Carcinoma, Clin. Immun. Immunopath. 10: 79
     (1978).
83. G. Sufrin, G.L. Tritsch, A. Mittelman and G.P. Murphy, Adenosine
     Deaminase Activity in Patients with Carcinoma of the Bladder,
     J. Urol. 119: 343 (1978).
84. M.D. Symes, H. Eckert, R.C.L. Feneley, T. Lai et al., Transfer
     of Adoptive Immunity by Intra-arterial Injection of Tumor Immune
     Pig Lymph Node Cells, Urology, 12: 398 (1978).
85. M. Takasugi, M.R. Mickey and P.I. Terasaki, Studies on Specifi-
     city of Cell Mediated Immunity to Human Tumors, J. Nat. Cancer
     Inst. 53: 1527 (1974).
86. T. Tanaka,E.H. Cooper and C.K. Anderson, Lymphocyte Infiltration
     in Bladder Carcinoma, Eur. J. Clin. Biol. Res. 15: 1085 (1970).
87. M. Troye, P. Perlmann, A. Larsson, H. Blomgren and B. Johansson,
     Cellular Toxicity in vitro in Transitional Cell Carcinoma.   Cr51
     Release Assay, Int. J. Cancer, 20: 188 (1977).
88. M. Troye, P. Perlmann, G.R. Pape, H.L. Spiegelberg, I. Näslund
     and A. Gidlöf, Use of Fab Fragments of Rabbit Anti-human Immuno-
     globulin as Analytic Tool for Establishing Involvement of
     Immunoglobulin in Spontaneous Cytotoxicity of Lymphocytes from
     Patients with Bladder Carcinomas, J. Immunol. 119: 1061 (1977).
89. G. Vermesse, D. Camus, P. Wattre, A. Capron and C. Gautier-Benoit
     Modifications Immunitaires dans les Suites Opératoires Immédiates
     N. Presse Med. 7: 529 (1978).
90. R.M. Vetto, D.R. Burger, A.A. Vandenbark and P.E. Finke, Changes
     in Tumor Immunity During Therapy Determined by Leucocyte Adher-
     ence Inhibition and Dermal Testing, Cancer, 41: 1034 (1978).
91. M. Vilien and H. Wolf, The Specificity of the Microcytotoxicity
     Assay for Cell-mediated Immunity in Human Bladder Cancer, J. Urol
     119: 338 (1978).
92. D. Viza, J. Phillips, C.L. Boucheix and F. Corrado, Associated
     Tumor Antigens in Leukemia, Melanoma and Lung Carcinoma,
     Franchimont - Cancer Related Antigens 77, Amsterdam (1976).
93. Z. Wajsman, C. Merrin, T.M. Chu, R.H. Moore and G.P. Murphy,
     Evaluation of Biological Markers in Bladder Cancer, J. Urol.
     114: 879 (1975).

94.   R.S. Weinstein, J. Alroy, G.M. Farrow, A.W. Miller and
      I. Davidsohn, Blood Group Isoantigen Deletion in Carcinoma in
      Situ of the Human Bladder, Cancer, 43: 661 (1979).
95.   A.K. Young, E. Hammond and A.W. Middleton, The Prognostic Value
      of Cell-surface Antigens in Low Grade, Non Invasive Transitional
      Cell Carcinoma of the Bladder, J. Urol. 122: 462 (1979).

CHEMOIMMUNE PROPHYLAXIS OF SUPERFICIAL BLADDER CANCER

H.D. ADOLPHS AND W. VAHLENSIECK

University Hospital
Bonn
Germany

INTRODUCTION

We developed the concept of chemoimmune prophylaxis on the basis of experimental findings. Since 1978 we have performed this treatment for prophylaxis of recurrence of superficial bladder cancer in our department.

Our own experimental work in rats showed that the induction and growth of experimental urinary bladder cancer can be significantly attenuated by BCG. This tumor protective effect becomes even more pronounced after pretreatment with cyclophosphamide (2, 3). Table 1 shows the inhibitory effect of both BCG and cyclophosphamide alone and in combination on the induction of bladder tumors in rats. To our knowledge, a synergistic effect of cyclophosphamide and BCG has not been shown before in experimental bladder cancer. However, there are other experimental cancer models which have already proved a definite synergistic action between chemotherapeutic agents and subsequent nonspecific immune stimulation (1, 2, 9, 12, 20, 21, 23, 25).

Method

We performed chemoimmune prophylaxis in 25 patients after complete resection of T1 urothelial bladder tumors by application of cyclophosphamide and BCG. Before starting this treatment, the following conditions had to be fulfilled:

1. The patient had to exhibit an intact cellular immune response as determined by a positive DNCB test. Fig. 1 shows a typical skin reaction 14 days after topical application of 2,000 µg DNCB on the arm.

Table 1
Effect of Cyclophosphamide, BCG and combined treatment on
experimental urinary bladder tumors.

Treatment	Bladder tumor weight (g)		Significant difference
	Median	Range	
CONTROL	3.1	3.2	-
CYCLOPHOSPHAMIDE	2.7	4.8	-
BCG	1.4	3.1	$p < 0.05$
CYCLOPHOSPHAMIDE + BCG	0.9	2.5	$p < 0.01$

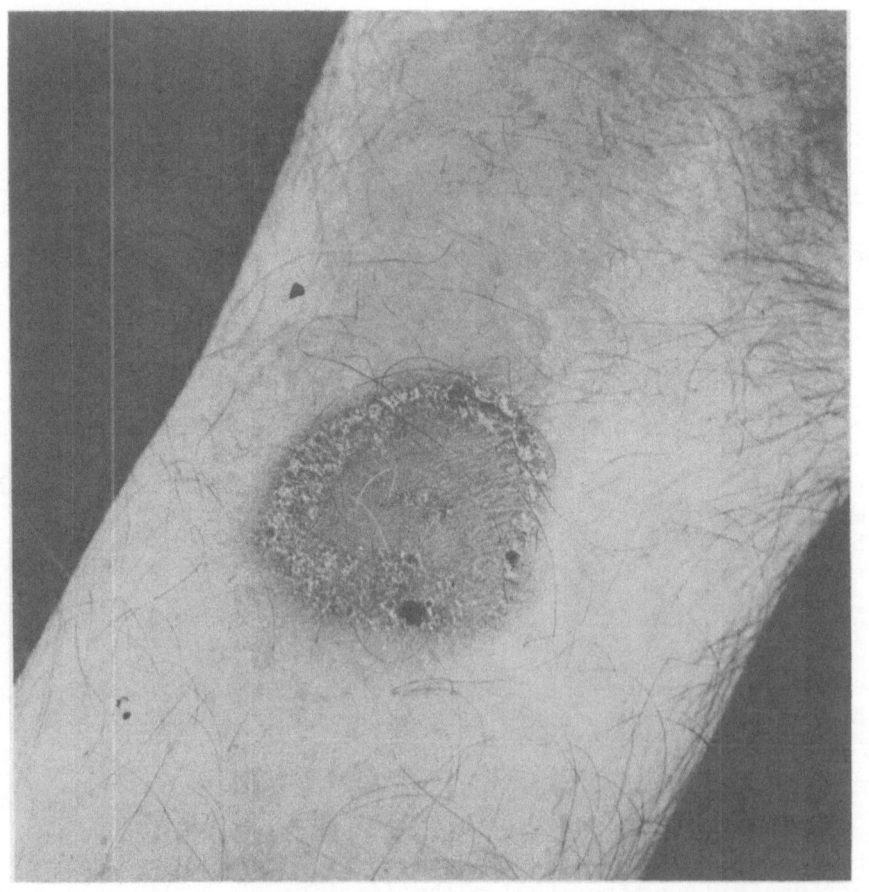

Fig. 1. Positive skin reaction after DNCB test.

2. The urine had to be free of bacterial infection.

Table 2 summarizes the treatment. On the 14th postoperative day, the patient received 700 mg Cyclophosphamide as a bolus intravenously. Two weeks later, 120 mg BCG (Connaught strain) was instilled in 50 ml saline intravesically by a catheter; the suspension was kept in the bladder for at least one hour. Simultaneously we performed a percu- taneous BCG immunisation on the right and left thigh, alternatively. BCG instillation together with skin scarification was repeated five times at weekly intervals. After termination of this treatment, the patient was assessed cytologically and endoscopically every three months. During the course of chemoimmune prophylaxis and later on, sporadic cold biopsies of the bladder mucosa were obtained and examin- ed histologically.

Results

Our results show that a recurrent tumor occured only in one case. All other patients remained tumor free within an observation period from 4 to 27 months (Table 3). At the beginning of the study we increased the number of patients only slowly for fear of possible side effects of BCG treatment Nine patients are presently followed more than 12 months. For comparison, after transurethral tumor resection

Table 2
Regimen for chemoimmune prophylaxis

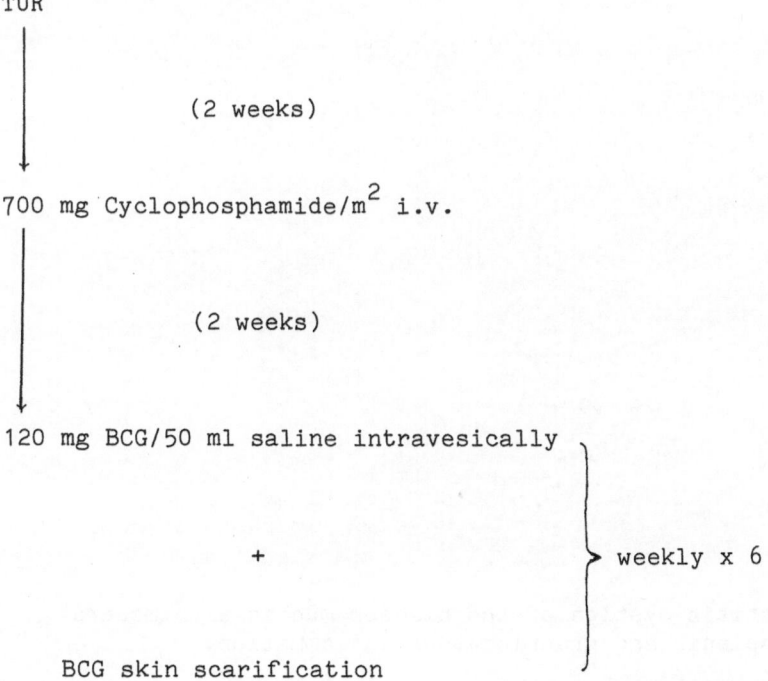

TUR

(2 weeks)

700 mg Cyclophosphamide/m^2 i.v.

(2 weeks)

120 mg BCG/50 ml saline intravesically

+   weekly x 6

BCG skin scarification

Table 3
Results of chemoimmune prophylaxis in 25 patients
with T1 GI-III tumors.

No. of Patients	Recurrence	Postoperative Time (Months)				
		0-6	7-12	13-18	19-24	>24
	No	9	6	3	3	3
25						
	Yes	1				

alone, our recurrence rates were 30% in the first year and 43% in the
second, under otherwise identical conditions. Side effects of this
treatment were well tolerated by the patients and essentially consisted of dysuria and transient mild fever; symptoms usually disappeared on the day after treatment. These preliminary results lead us
to the conclusion that chemoimmune prophylaxis might be effective in
preventing tumor recurrences.

During and after topical BCG treatment, the bladder mucosa
underwent the typical changes of chronic inflammation. Histologically the picture of cystitis cystica with moderate urothelial
dysplasia and granulomatous inflammation was predominant (Fig. 2).

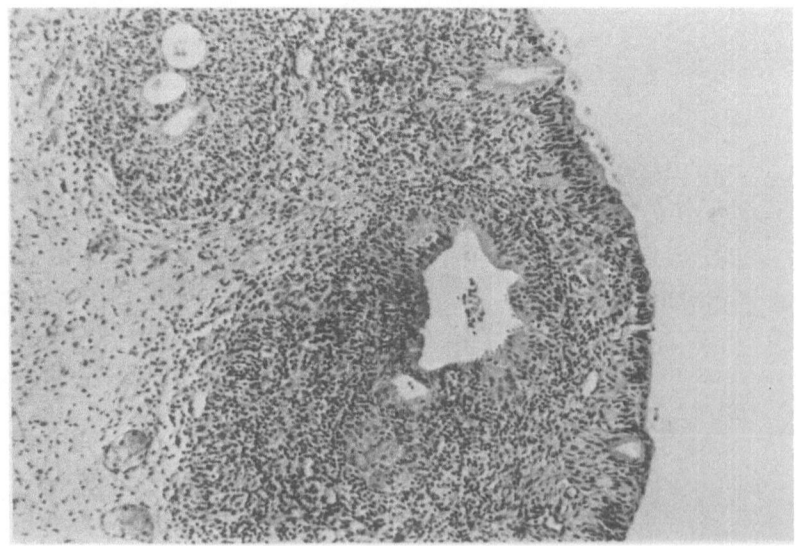

Fig. 2.   Cystitis cystica of the bladder mucosa with moderate
          dysplasia and granulomatous inflammation.

A higher magnification illustrates a typical granuloma consisting of epithelioid and giant cells with surrounding lymphocytic inflammation (Fig. 3).

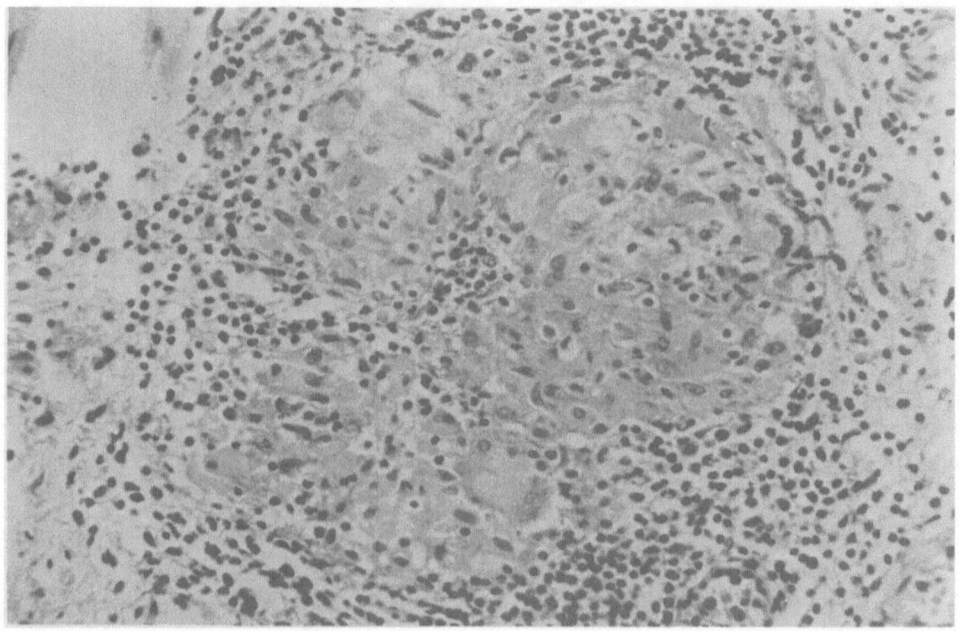

Fig. 3. Epithelioid and giant cells with surrounding lymphocytic inflammation of the bladder mucosa.

Sometimes dypslastic changes became so marked that transition into carcinoma in situ was evident (Fig. 4).

Three months after termination of BCG treatment, the mucosa was endoscopically normal without any major histological alterations.

DISCUSSION

Martinez-Piñeiro and Muntañola (17) and Morales et al. (18) were able to demonstrate a favourable tumor protective effect in a few patients after intravesical BCG application. Lamm et al. (15) were the first to prove the value of topical BCG prophylaxis in a prospective randomized study. The results showed a statistically significant favourable effect on the recurrence rate in the BCG treated group compared with no treatment. In this study, however, no cyclophosphamide was given.

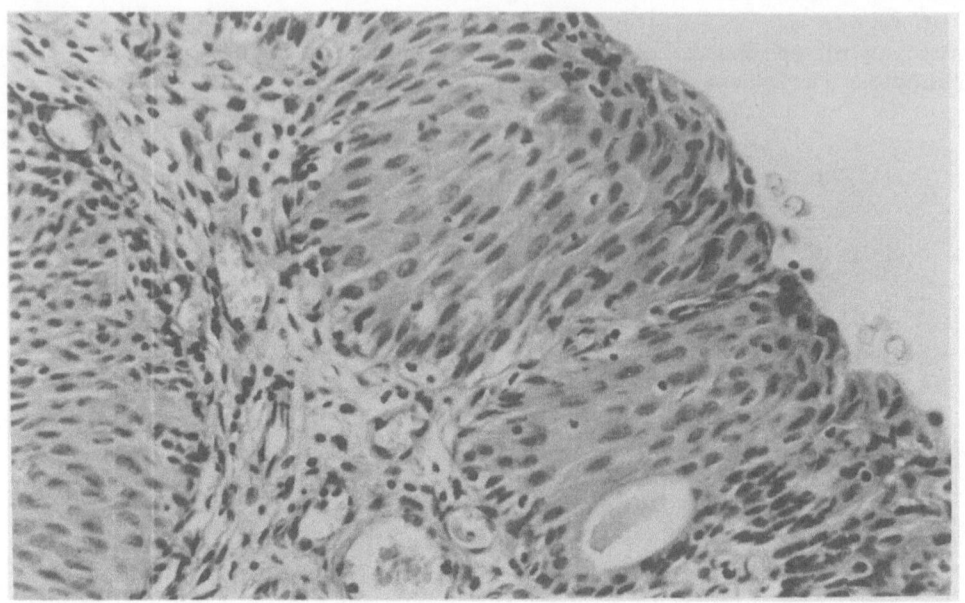

Fig. 4.   Carcinoma in situ like lesion of the bladder mucosa.

        As far as the mode of action of cyclophosphamide and BCG
treatment is concerned, experimental evidence has been obtained
that:

1.   Cyclophosmphaide leads to suppression of humoral immune response
     and consequently to a decrease of immune complex formation
     (7,14,16,19).

2.   Cyclophosphamide effects a stimulation of cellular immune
     response by inhibition of suppressor cell precursors (4,8,10,13,
     22,24).

3.   BCG exerts a nonspecific stimulation of cellular immune response
     (11,26).

        More clinical research has to be done in order to find out to
what extent these immunological mechanisms are also effective in
patients.

REFERENCES

1.   H.D. Adolphs and L. Steffens, Theoretische und praktische
     Möglichkeiten der Immuntherapie maligner urologischer Tumoren,
     Helv. chir. Acta 43: 285 (1976).
2.   H.D. Adolphs, J. Thiele, and H. Kiel, Effect of Intralesional

and Systemic BCG-application or a combined Cyclophosphamide/BCG Treatment on Experimental Bladder Cancer, Urol. Res. 7: 71 (1979).

3. H.D. Adolphs, J. Thiele, and H. Kiel, Inhibition of Experimental Bladder Tumor Induction by Systemic BCG Treatment, Eur. Urol. In Press.

4. P.W. Askenase, B.J. Hayden, and R.K. Gershon, Augmentation of delayed type hypersensitivity by doses of Cyclophosphamide which do not Affect Antibody Responses, J. exp. Med. 141: 697 (1975).

5. R.C. Bast, Jr., B. Zbar, T. Borsos, and H.J. Rapp, BCG and cancer (first of two parts), N. Engl. J. Med. 290: 1413 (1974).

6. R.C. Bast, Jr., B. Zbar, T. Borsos, and H.J. Rapp, BCG and Cancer (second of two parts), N. Engl. J. Med. 290: 1458 (1974).

7. H.H. Buskirk, J.A. Crim, H.G. Petering, K. Merritt, and A.G. Johnson, Effect of Uracil Mustard and Several Antitumor Drugs on the Primary Antibody Response in Rats and Mice, J. Nat. Cancer Inst. 34: 747 (1965).

8. R.M. Ferguson and R.L. Simmons, Differential Cyclophosphamide Sensitivity of Suppressor and Cytotoxic Cell Percusors, Transplantation 25: 36 (1978).

9. B. Fisher, H. Rubin, E. Saffer, and N. Wolmark, The Effect of Corynebacterium Parvum in Combination with 5-Fluorouracil, L-Phenylalanine Mustard, or Methotrexate on the Inhibition of Tumor Growth, Cancer Res. 36: 2714 (1976).

10. H.K. Gill and F.Y. Liew, Regulation of Delayed-type Hypersensitivity. III. Effect of Cyclophosphamide on the Suppressor Cells for Delayed-type Hypersensitivity to Sheep Erythrocytes in Mice, Eur. J. Immunol. 8: 172 (1978).

11. J.U. Gutterman, G. Mavligit, C. McBride, E. Frei III, and E.M. Hersh, Immunoprophylaxis of Malignant Melanoma with Systemic BCG: Study of Strain, Dose and Schedule. Nat. Cancer Inst. Monograph No.' 39: 205 (1973).

12. T. Hattori and S. Yamagata, Combined Treatment with Anaerobic Corynebacterium Liquefaciens and Chemotherapeutics against Solid Tumor in Mice, Gann. 68: 115 (1977).

13. M. Hurme, Differential Cyclophosphamide Sensitivity of Precursor Cells in Allogeneic and H.2 Restricted Cytotoxic Responses, J. exp. Med. 149: 290 (1979).

14. S. Husberg, H. Ericsson, Influence of Cyclophosphamide on the Antibody Response Evoked by an Experimental Sarcoma in Rats, Transplantation 26: 135 (1978).

15. D.L. Lamm, D.E. Thor, S.C. Harris, J.A. Reyna, V.D. Stogdill, and H.M. Radwin, BCG Immunotherapy of Superficial Bladder Cancer, J. Urol. 124: 38 (1980).

16. S.P. Lerman and W.P. Weidanz, The Effect of Cyclophosphamide on the Ontogeny of the Humoral Immune Response in Chickens, J. Immunol. 105: 614 (1970).

17. J.A. Martinez-Piñeiro and P. Muntañola, Nonspecific Immunotherapy with BCG Vaccine in Bladder Tumors. A Preliminary Report. Eur. Urol. 3: 11 (1977).

18. A. Morales, D. Eidinger, and A.W. Bruce, Intracavitary
    Bacillus Calmette-Guerin in the Treatment of Superficial
    Bladder Tumors, J. Urol. 116: 180 (1976).
19. I.G. Otterness and Y.H. Shang, Comparative Study of
    Cyclophosphamide, 6-Mercaptopurine, Azathiopurine and
    Methotrexate, Clin. exp. Immunol. 26: 346 (1976).
20. D.M. Purnell, G.L. Bartlett, J.W. Kreider, and T.G. Biro,
    Corynebacterium parvum and Cyclophsphamide as Combination
    Treatment for a Murine Mammary Adenocarcinoma, Cancer Res.
    37: 1137 (1977).
21. W.A. Sansing, J.J. Killion, and G.M. Kollmorgen, Evaluation of
    Time and Dose in Treating Mammary Adenocarcinoma with
    Immunostimulants, Cancer Immunol. Immunother. 2: 63 (1977).
22. A. Schwartz, P.W. Askenase, and R.K. Gershon, Regulation of
    Delayed-type Hypersensitivity Reactions by Cyclophosphamide-
    sensitive T cells, J. Immunol. 121: 1573 (1978).
23. M.T. Scott, Analysis of the Principles Underlying Chemo-
    immunotherapy of Mouse Tumours. I. Treatment with
    Cyclophosphamide Followed by Corynebacterium Parvum,
    Cancer Immunol. Immunother. 6: 107 (1979).
24. M.S. Sy, S.D. Miller, and H.N. Claman, Immune Suppression
    with Supraoptimal Doses of Antigen in Contact Sensitivity.
    I. Demonstration of Suppressor Cells and their Sensitivty
    to Cyclophosphamide, J. Immunol. 119: 240 (1977).
25. A. Tagliabue, N. Polentarutti, A Vecchi, A. Mantovani, and
    F. Spreafico, Combination Chemo-immunotherapy with Adriamycin
    in Experimental Tumor Systems, Eur. J. Cancer 13: 657 (1977).
26. B. Zbar, E. Ribi, M. Kelly, D. Granger, C. Evans, and H.J. Rapp,
    Immunologic Approaches to the Treatment of Human Cancer Based
    on a Guinea Pig Model, Cancer Immunol. Immunother. 1: 127 (1976).

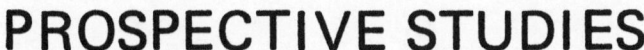

PROSPECTIVE STUDIES

CHAIRMAN'S SUMMARY

L ANDERSSON
Department of Urology, Karolinska sjukhuset
Stockholm, Sweden

The development in recent years of cancer chemotherapy and of
multimodal therapy in malignant diseases has been based mainly on
empirical experience. It would be desirable to have in vitro tests
of the sensitivity or resistance of the tumour cells to various
cytostatic agents analogous to sensitivity tests in bacterial infec-
tions. Tissue culture of bladder carcinoma is now possible and some
investigators have even studied the reaction of tumour cells following exposure to cytostatic drugs. So far, however, the reproducibility of such resistance tests has been unsatisfactory and often
the growth inhibition in vitro has not been paralleled in the patient.
Prospective trials under controlled conditions still remain our most
important instrument to investigate the efficacy of cancer chemotherapy.

In carcinoma of the bladder, as in prostate cancer, chemotherapy is still much less successful than in a number of other
tumours, e.g. carcinoma of the testis. Even though improved results
have recently been reported, at least in the treatment of bladder
carcinoma, intensified research is urgently needed.

Few, if any, institutions have at their disposal enough
patients to perform, on their own and within a reasonable period
of time, a randomised chemotherapy trial which would permit even
subgrouping according to tumour grade and stage. It is preferable
to perform such trials on a multicentre basis. On the other hand
multicentre co-operation implies a number of difficulties, the most
serious being inconsistencies in recording progression and, even
more, regression of deep tissue tumours. We hope that new techniques,
such as transvesical or transrectal ultrasonotomography and computed
axial tomography, will be helpful for the objective measurement of

tumour mass. More experience is needed before we can judge the true
value of these new techniques. Estimation of the degree of infiltration of a bladder or prostatic carcinoma by palpation is very
inaccurate. Reduction of tumour infiltration by at least 50% is a
common criterion of partial therapy response but using methods of
measurement available today, all such estimations imply an element
of subjective judgement.

We know from experience that uniform evaluation of deep tumours
is difficult to accomplish and can vary within one and the same
centre with different investigators. This difficulty becomes even
greater in multicentric studies and some critics reject such trials
as of no real value. It is quite evident, however, that a number of
well organised multicentric trials, national or international, have
contributed significantly to our present knowledge of chemotherapy
and multimodal therapy in cancer.

To provide adequate information a multicentric study, like a
monocentric study, must, of course, keep within a strictly defined
protocol designed to clearly establish, among other things, the
tumour category, the criteria for progression and regression, and
the indications of failure of treatment.

In practice these ideals cannot always be met. Optimal co-
operation implies frequent communication with regular conferences
between the participating centres and perhaps even mutual reminders
and encouragement. Many of the drawbacks hampering multicentric
trials can be compensated by a sufficiently solid organisation and
good personal contacts between the participants.

INTRAVESICAL CHEMOPROPHYLAXIS OF SUPERFICIAL BLADDER CANCER

H RÜBBEN and W LUTZEYER

Department of Urology
Rheinisch-Westfälisch Technischen Hochschule
Aachen, West Germany

Prospective studies concerning therapy of malignant diseases are supported by the German Government - Bundesregierung für Forschung und Technologie, - BMFT -. These studies of urinary tract tumors are coordinated by the department of Urology and Pathology of the Rheinisch-Westfälisch Technischen Hochschule - RWTH - Aachen.

Up to now there are two protocols concerning intravesical chemoprophylaxis of superficial bladder cancer after complete transurethral resection. The reason for preparing these two protocols is summarized as follows:

Approximately 60% of superficial bladder tumors removed by transurethral resection, open excision or open resection recur (1,2, 3,5,6,9,18). Lymph node metastases are expected in less than 10% in the tumor categories Ta and T1 and distant metastases are an infrequent complication in the follow up of superficial bladder cancer (4,8,11,15,16).

The frequency of the tumor categories according to the stage and the grade of the urothelial tumors is depicted in Table 1 (14, 17). The most frequent tumor (24%) is the well differentiated non invasive carcinoma (TaG1). Ta and T1 tumors are understaged by clinical examination, biopsy, bimanual palpation and diagnostic transurethral resection in 12% and T2 tumors in 31% of the cases (Table 2).

The three year survival rate of patients with transitional cell carcinoma shows a strong correlation to the grade and the stage of the tumor (Table 3).

TABLE 1

Percentage frequency of urothelial bladder carcinomas
according to stage and grade (n = 900)

T/G	1	2	3
a	24	4	1
1	11	15	2
2	3	8	5
3	-	5	8
4	-	2	4

TaG0 5%, dysplasia 2%, undifferentiated carcinoma 1%.

TABLE 2

Incidence or clinical understaging (n=290)

T	histopathological diagnosis a/1	2	3	4	understaging (per cent)
clinical diagnosis					
a/1	207	22	6	-	12
2	11	27	10	7	31

clinical: biopsy, bimanual palpation, diagnostic TUR
histological: definitive histological diagnosis of the specimen

TABLE 3

Three year survival rate of superficial transitional cell
carcinomas according to stage and grade in % (n = 315)

T/G	1	2	3
a	97	90	-
1	92	72	57
2	-	53	27

Superficial bladder carcinomas are multifocal tumors in 30%; the incidence in category Ta, T1 or T2 lesions being very similar at 28%, 35% and 23% respectively (n=315). However the incidence of multiple tumors does vary considerably. Primary Ta and T1 tumors show multifocal tumor growth in 25% only, whereas 45% of recurrent Ta and T1 tumors are multifocal (n=274).

The overall percentage of tumors which recur within three years is 64%. The recurrence rate is influenced greatly by stage but only slightly by grade. Ta tumors are followed by a recurrence in 52%, T1 in 69%, T2 in 77%, G1 in 63%, G2 in 67% and G3 in 71% of the cases (n=315). The frequency of recurrence further depends on whether the lesion is primary or recurrent. 45% of primary tumors recur, the first recurrence being followed by a second recurrence in 84%. These findings do not depend on the higher percentage of worse differentiated or infiltrative tumors in the group of recurrences and can be observed even when TaG1 or TaG2 tumor categories only are considered (Table 4).

In the same manner the frequency of recurrence is also influenced by the presence or absence of multifocal tumors. Solitary superficial tumors recur in 46%, multifocal tumors in 73%; the figures concerning TaG1 tumors only are 29% (solitary) and 94% (multifocal) (Table 5).

Tumor progression depends on the grade and the stage of the primary tumor. Ta tumors recur in a higher grade or stage in 19%, T1 in 34%, T2 in 46%, G1 tumors in 20%, G2 in 37% and G3 in 64%.

The interval between the primary tumor and the recurrence of higher grade or stage is influenced by the differentiation and also by the depth of infiltration of the primary tumor. TaG1 tumors show tumor progression in about two years, T1G2 tumors in 14 months and T2G3 tumors in less than one year (Table 6).

TABLE 4

Percentage of recurrences after TUR, open resection or excision of the primary tumor and of the first recurrence

	primary tumor	first recurrence	
Ta - T2	45	84	(n=315)
TaG1	42	85	
TaG2	55	75	(n=185)

TABLE 5

Percentage of recurrences after TUR, open resection or excision
of solitary and multifocal tumors

	solitary	multifocal	
Ta - T2	46	73	(n = 315)
primary TaG1	29	94	(n = 120)
primary TaG2	50	(3/3)	

Noninvasive tumors show tumor progression in 20% (primary) and
25% (recurrent) respectively. But the percentage of progression is
very different in T1 primary and recurrent tumors; the figures are
24% and 56% respectively. In the same manner figures are different
when comparing solitary and multifocal tumors (Table 7).

As yet there are only four published reports of randomized
studies. In three of these studies, involving instillation therapy,
Thiotepa has been used (3,10,13). Although there was a small
reduction of the recurrence rate intravesical chemoprophylaxis with
Thiotepa was not shown to be of great value at the dosage and
instillation interval used. The study of Jacobi (7) who instilled
Adriamycin includes only 15 treated patients and therefore there
are no statistically significant results as yet.

There are at least three more protocols active at the moment:
EORTC Protocol 30782: Thiotepa vs Adriamycin vs Cisplatinum
"Innsbruck, München, Mainz": Mitomycin C vs Adriamycin vs VM-26
EORTC Protocol 30790: Adriamycin vs Epodyl vs TUR only.

TABLE 6

Interval in months between primary tumor and recurrence of
higher grade or stage

T/G	1	2	3
a	23.5		
1		14.5	14.0
2		14.2	10.2

(n = 315)

TABLE 7

Percentage of tumors with recurrence of
higher grade or stage (n=274)

	primary	recurrent	solitary	multiple
Ta	20	25	18	43
T1	24	56	33	46

The first two protocols will probably show that one of the tested drugs is superior but will not be able to show that chemoprophylaxis is of definite value. The third protocol, EORTC protocol 30790, includes a control group - i.e. no further therapy after transurethral resection. In this protocol chemoprophylaxis starts not earlier than 14 days after transurethral resection. The first results of this study are expected in about three years.

On the basis of these active protocols and the data mentioned above our protocols have been prepared as follows:

"B M F T - Adriamycin": The first instillation is performed immediately before transurethral resection to reduce the implantation of exfoliated tumor cells in the mucosa traumatized during the transurethral resection. Histologically diagnosed Ta and T1 tumors, G1 to G3, (17) are then randomized to receive either:

i. no further therapy
ii. instillation therapy twice weekly for six weeks, or
iii. instillation therapy twice weekly for six weeks, twice monthly for 4.5. months and once monthly for six months.

At each instillation 50 mg Adriamycin is dissolved in 50 ml physiologic saline solution and instilled for two hours. The aim of this study is to answer two questions:

i. Is Adriamycin able to reduce the frequency of recurrences or tumor progression in general?
ii. Is a short perioperative regimen sufficient or is long term instillation therapy necessary?

"B M F T - Mitomycin C", the second study, also involves instillation just before transurethral resection. After randomization the patient receives Mitomycin C 20 mg in 20 ml distilled water in one of the following regimens:

i. twice weekly for six weeks, twice monthly for 4.5 months and once monthly for six months,

ii. twice weekly for six weeks, then once monthly for 20.5 months,
iii. twice weekly for six weeks and after that once every second
month for 20.5 months.

The aim of this study is to determine the interval between the
instillation dates which is necessary to guarantee the usefulness
of the instillation therapy.

In both protocols tumors are stratified as primary or
recurrent.

These studies will be evaluated by the frequency of recurrences,
the recurrence rate, the interval between the first treated tumor
and the next recurrence, the percentage of tumor progression, the
percentage of multifocal tumor growth and by the percentage of
dysplastic areas in the microscopically normal mucosa, assessed by
random biopsies which have to be performed in all patients at the
start and at the end of the study, four years after the first
instillation. So far only 60 patients have been entered into these
protocols and therefore no results are yet available.

REFERENCES

1. R. Barnes, H. Hadley, A. Dick, Johnson, J. Dexter, Changes in
grade and stage of recurrent bladder tumors, J. Urol. 118: 177
(1977).
2. R.W. Barnes, R.T. Bergmann, H.C. Hadley, D. Love, Control of
bladder tumors by endoscopic surgery, J. Urol. 97: 864 (1967).
3. D. Byar, C. Blackard and VACURG, Comparison of placebo,
pyridoxine and topical thiotepa in preventing recurrence of stage I
bladder cancer, Urology 10: 556 (1977).
4. C.I. Cooling, Review of 150 post-mortems of carcinoma of the
urinary bladder, in: "Tumours of the bladder. Neoplastic diseases
at various sites. Vol 2." D.M. Wallace, ed., E. & S. Livingstone Ltd,
Edinburgh 171, Baltimore, The Williams & Wilkins Company (1959).
5. H.A. Gilbert, J.L. Logan, A.R. Kagan, H.A. Friedman, J.K. Cove,
M. Fox, T.M. Muldoon, Y.M. Lonni, J.H. Rowe, J.F. Cooper, H. Nussbaum,
P. Chain, A. Rao, A. Starr, The natural history of papillary transitional cell carcinoma of the bladder and its treatment in an
unselected population on the basis of histologic grading, J. Urol.
119: 488 (1978).
6. F.L. Greene, K.A. Hanash and G.M. Farrow, Benign papilloma or
papillary carcinoma of the bladder, J.Urol. 110: 205 (1973).
7. G.H. Jacobi, K.H. Kurth, K.F. Klippel and R. Hohenfellner, On
the biological behaviour of T1-transitional cell tumors of the
urinary bladder and initial results of prophylactic use of topical
adriamycin under controlled and randomized conditions, WHO
Collaborating Centre for Research and Treatment of Urinary Bladder
Cancer, Stockholm, p 83 (September 1978).

8. H.J. Jewett and G.H. Strong, Infiltrating carcinoma of the
bladder: Relation of depth of penetration of the bladder wall to
incidence of local extension and metastases, J. Urol. 55: 366 (1946).
9. A. Miller, J.P. Mitchell and N.J. Brown, The Bristol bladder
tumor registry. Brit. J. Urol. 41 (Suppl.):1 (1969).
10. P.T. Nieh, J.J. Daly, J.A. Heaney, N.M. Heney and G.R. Prout.
The effect of thiotepa on normal and tumor epithelium, J. Urol.
119: 59 (1978).
11. J.P. Richie, D.G. Skinner and J.J. Kaufman, Radical cystectomy
for carcinoma of the bladder: 16 years of experience, J. Urol.
113: 186 (1975).
12. H. Rübben, H.H. Dahm, V.W. Uelft and W. Lutzeyer, TNM-
Klassifikation maligner Blasentumoren UICC 1979. Arbeitsgrundlage
des "Registers und Verbundstudie für Harnwegstumoren RWTH Aachen",
Urologe A 18: 1 (1979).
13. C. Schulman, R. Sylvester, M. Robinson, P. Smith, A. Lachand,
L. Denis, M. Pavone-Macaluso, M. de Pauw, and M. Staquet, Adjuvant
therapy of T1 bladder carcinoma: Preliminary results of an EORTC
randomized study, in: "Recent Results in Cancer Research Vol 68."
G. Bonadonna, G. Mathe and S.E. Salmon, eds., Springer-Verlag,
Berlin (1979).
14. UICC: TNM classification of malignant tumors, M.H. Harmer, ed.,
3rd edition, Imprimerie G. de Buren S.A., Geneve (1978).
15. H.E. Walther, Krebsmetastasen, Schwabe und Co., Basel (1948).
16. Z. Wajsman, G. Baumgartner, G.P. Murphy and C. Merrin,
Evaluation of lymphangiography for clinical staging of bladder
tumors, J. Urol. 114: 712 (1975).
17. WHO: World Health Organization. Histological typing of
urinary bladder tumors, in: "International Histological Classification of Tumors," Geneva (1973).
18. H. Zincke, Das Blasenkarzinom, in: "Verhandlungsbericht der
Deutschen Gesellschaft für Urologie," Springer-Verlag, Berlin and
Heidelberg.

PROSPECTIVE STUDIES OF THE EORTC UROLOGICAL GROUP

P H SMITH

Department of Urology
St. James's University Hospital
Leeds, England

INTRODUCTION

The Urological Group of the EORTC (European Organisation for the Research on the Treatment of Cancer) was formed in 1975. At that time we discussed the contribution that we should attempt to make to the management of patients with bladder cancer and concluded that there were two main objectives:-

1.   to evaluate intravesical chemotherapy in category T1 bladder cancer and

2.   to contribute to the search for effective cytotoxic regimes for patients with invasive bladder cancer.

It is the results of the early studies and our current views that I should like to present to you today.

CHEMOTHERAPY IN SUPERFICIAL BLADDER CANCER

At least 70% of category Ta/T1 bladder tumours recur following transurethral resection (TUR) and, in 10% of such patients, recurrence shows a higher T or G category (4). In addition, it is increasingly recognised that carcinoma in situ may be found in patients with superficial tumours. The problems presented by recurrence, progression and carcinoma in situ demand detailed evaluation of intravesical chemotherapy and of other treatments which may be used following TUR.

Dr. Schulman has already reported the results of our first study (Protocol 30751) which demonstrated the superiority of

intravesical Thiotepa over VM-26 and no additional treatment in
reducing the recurrence rate following transurethral resection of
category T1 bladder cancer. Whilst planning our subsequent studies
it soon became apparent that, although many drugs had been used for
intravesical chemotherapy, information on large numbers of patients
was available only for Adriamycin, Epodyl and Thiotepa (15).

Adriamycin

It is known that Adriamycin is found in maximal concentration
in the liver and lymph nodes following intravenous injection (7);
there is also selective uptake in bladder cancers for periods in
excess of six hours following a single intravenous injection of
60 mg (10).

The treatment schedule used for intravesical administration
has varied greatly, the dose ranging from 10 to 100 mgs, concentration from 0.33 to 2 mg per ml, time of exposure from one to two
hours, the volume of administration from 20 ml to a volume of 50 ml
short of the bladder capacity and the frequency of admission from
daily for a fortnight to once a month. It has also been shown that
a dosage of 50 mg or more is required to give the best chance of
remission and it is this dose of 50 mg which we have chosen for our
studies (3,6,8).

Epodyl

Riddle has extensive experience with Epodyl (11,12) and has
demonstrated that complete and partial remissions are likely to be
seen in over half the patients but that if treatment is continued
for three years remission will be complete or recurrence will have
occurred. In analysing the long term follow up of these patients
he observed that, in the event of a complete and sustained remission,
death from bladder cancer was most unlikely, whilst after complete
remission followed by relapse or in the event of partial remission
or no response, death from bladder cancer was the most probable
outcome. Although he used Epodyl with minimal toxicity, the
experience of the Yorkshire Urological Cancer Research Group (YUCRG)
was less satisfactory (13) in that although complete or partial
remission was seen in 37 of 51 patients, remission was unlikely to
occur in patients with poorly differentiated lesions and was
associated with significant toxicity, this being seen in 30 of 51
patients; cystitis and subsequent bladder contracture occurred in
10 patients, leading to the necessity for cystectomy and urinary
diversion in two.

Thiotepa

This agent has been the most commonly used in the last twenty
years and we have found few problems with it. Despite the fact

that its molecular weight (M.Wt.) of 189 is lower than that of Epodyl (M.Wt. 262) and of Adriamycin (M.Wt. 580) we have seen little evidence of systemic toxicity (Table 1) and we regard this agent as the reference drug against which others are to be judged.

Treatment Schedules

We considered the desirability of immediate and of delayed administration of the agents. It is obviously easiest to carry out the administration at the time of TUR but this may increase local and systemic toxicity. Because of this we decided to instil the agents up to thirty days following TUR in our first study. In one replacement study (Protocol 30782) the time of administration chosen is within three days or between 10 and 14 days. This should allow us to obtain further information on the toxicity of the agents administered very shortly following TUR.

As we were developing our new intravesical studies we were much interested in the paper by Byar et al (1) in which 121 patients were randomised to receive oral Pyridoxine, intravesical Thiotepa or no additional treatment following transurethral resection of category T1 bladder tumours. This study showed some evidence that Pyridoxine might reduce the chance of recurrence if given on a regular and prolonged basis.

Our eventual decision was to implement three studies, all of which are now active. Of these, two involve intravesical chemotherapy and the third the oral use of Pyridoxine and Placebo on a double blind basis following complete TUR for Ta/T1 bladder cancer.

1.   Protocol 30781 (Study Coordinators Mr. M.R.G. Robinson, Pontefract, and Mr. D. Newling, Hull, United Kingdom).

In this study patients with category Ta/T1 bladder cancer are treated with Pyridoxine or Placebo on a double blind basis after complete resection of all visible lesions. At the time of diagnosis, and after six months of treatment, tryptophan metabolites are investigated before and after a tryptophan load test. The patient takes one tablet each day, which may be Pyridoxine 20 mg or Placebo and at each check cystoscopy (every three months in the first year and not less than six-monthly thereafter) blood is sent to Roche Laboratories in Basle for assessment of pyridoxal phosphate and asparate amino transferase.

So far this study has recruited 157 of the 186 evaluable patients required, all from the United Kingdom.

2.   Protocol 30782 (Study Coordinators Dr. C.C. Schulman, Brussels, Belgium and Professor M. Pavone-Macaluso, Palermo, Italy) is restricted to patients with recurrent category Ta/T1 bladder cancer

TABLE 1

HAEMATOLOGICAL TOXICITY IN EORTC PROTOCOL 30751

(FROM INTERIM ANALYSIS OF THIS STUDY CARRIED OUT ON 18.9.78)

TOXICITY	THIOTEPA (89 PATIENTS)	VM-26 (84 PATIENTS)	NO TREATMENT (82 PATIENTS)
WBC's < 4,500	2	3	2
PLATELETS < 150,000	14	16	10
WBC < 4,500 AND PLATELETS < 150,000	4	3	–
HAEMOGLOBIN < 11gms/100ml	1	1	2
HAEMOGLOBIN < 11gms/100ml AND WBC < 4,500	1	–	–
HAEMOGLOBIN < 11gms/100ml AND PLATELETS < 150,000	–	–	2
T O T A L	22	23	16

and compares the effect of Adriamycin 50 mg $_{vs}$ Cis Platinum 50 mg
vs Thiotepa 50 mg upon tumour free interval, recurrence rate and
incidence of increase of T or G category after complete resection
of all visible lesions. The drug allocated by randomisation is
instilled either within the first three days after transurethral
resection or between 10 and 14 days after TUR. It is then given
weekly for four weeks and monthly for eleven months. This study
now contains 124 of the 279 evaluable patients required, mostly
entered by surgeons from Belgium and France.

3.   Protocol 30790 (Study Coordinator Dr. K. Kurth, Rotterdam,
The Netherlands).

In this study Adriamycin 50 mg is compared with Epodyl 100 ml
1.13% and with no additional treatment following complete resection
of all visible lesions in patients with primary and recurrent
category Ta/T1 lesions. Patients are stratified into those with
primary and with recurrent lesions and those with single and with
multiple tumours. The treatment regime is similar to that in the
other intravesical studies. The first instillation must be carried
out within 14 days of TUR. Forty-eight of the 279 evaluable
patients required have so far been entered, largely from Holland
and Germany.

Having been involved with these studies for the last five
years, I am increasingly convinced that this form of therapy is of
potential value and requires further evaluation, not only to find
out which drugs are the most effective but also to refine the
techniques of administration by determining the ideal dose, concentration and volume of infusion, duration of exposure to the drug,
and frequency of administration.

It must be accepted that such treatment is inconvenient for
the patient who must attend repeatedly, that infective or chemical
cystitis may occur and that, theoretically at least, absorption of
the drug may lead to systemic toxicity. In the doses used however
this last complication is exceedingly unlikely. However, when one
considers that 80% of superficial tumours recur, up to 30% have
associated carcinoma in situ (14) and that at least 10% progress
to higher stage or higher grade (4) the need for effective treatment
is obvious. This attitude has recently been reinforced by the
observations of Murphy and Soloway (9) that intravesical chemotherapy, at least in mice, is associated with a lower incidence of
development of high grade and high stage lesions in the FANFT tumour
model and that such treatment may delay the progression of low
grade to high grade lesions.

CHEMOTHERAPY IN INVASIVE BLADDER CANCER

The early death rate in patients with invasive bladder cancer
is very high, 40% being dead after one year, whether treated by
cystectomy, radiotherapy alone or in combination with cystectomy (16).
Many of these patients die with metastases and it seems clear that
invasive bladder cancer in at least 40% of patients is not confined
to the pelvis at the time of diagnosis. These results emphasise the
need for some other form of treatment. The only logical approach at
the moment appears to be by means of systemic chemotherapy. At the
time that our Urological Group was formed we determined to carry out
a series of Phase II studies with the aim of developing a successful
regime to use in the adjuvant situation. We chose the combination
of Adriamycin 50 mg/m^2 and 5FU 500 mg/m^2 on a three weekly basis for
our first study which has previously been reported (5) and which
showed an objective remission rate of 40%. At this stage we were
uncertain whether the Adriamycin or the 5FU was the effective agent
and decided to implement a comparative Phase II study to compare
Adriamycin 75 mg/m^2, Adriamycin and 5FU in the doses given above
and Cyclophosphamide 1 gm/m^2 to obtain further information and to
evaluate Cyclophosphamide. Unfortuantely this study did not generate
sufficient interest and was closed to entry after eighteen months.

In 1978 we activated additional Phase II studies. The first
was designed to obtain further information on the combination of
Cyclophosphamide, Adriamycin and Cis Platinum and was the priority
study; the second, for those not eligible for entry to this protocol,
involved a Phase II assessment of Vincristine.

1.   Protocol 30771 (Study Coordinator Dr. E.J.H. Mulder, Rotterdam,
The.Netherlands).

In this study Cyclophosphamide, Adriamycin and Cis Platinum
were administered at doses of 400, 40 and 40 mg/m^2 respectively
every three weeks with evaluation after two cycles of therapy. Of
40 evaluable patients, remission was seen in 35% (complete remission
in three patients, partial remission in 11 patients, stable disease
in 21 patients and progression in five patients). Full details of
this study are now being prepared for publication.

2.   Protocol 30797 (Study Coordinator Mr. B. Richards, York,
United Kingdom).

This study has now recruited 21 evaluable patients. Remissions
of the primary lesions in the bladder have been seen in three
patients (complete in 1 and partial in 2). This study continues.

Our next study will evaluate the combination of Cis Platinum
70 mg/m^2 on Day 1 and VM26 100 mg/m^2 on Days 1 and 2 in three
weekly cycles.

Recruitment to these Phase II studies has so far been slow, in part because of urological inertia which now seems to be decreasing and in part because many of the patients are elderly and are not suitable for the more intensive forms of treatment.

Justification for such therapy lies in the symptomatic relief which undoubtedly occurs in these patients with advanced disease irrespective of the presence or absence of objective remission (2) and in the hope that the regimen which appears to be most active will be effective in the adjuvant situation. The EORTC Urological Group has now implemented an adjuvant study which is outlined below.

EORTC Protocol 30784 (Study Coordinator Professor Martinez-Pineiro, Madrid, Spain).

In this study patients with category P3 N0-2 M0 bladder cancer are randomly allocated to chemotherapy with Adriamycin and 5FU or no additional therapy after completion of primary treatment. Centres are allowed to chose between cystectomy, and preoperative radiotherapy (1500 rads in two days) followed by cystectomy in two to five days, as the primary treatment and are expected to adhere to the same primary treatment throughout the trial. The patient is eligible for the trial if at cystectomy the lesion is category P3 N0-2 M0. Randomisation is carried out after successful completion of the primary treatment. However if patients have not recovered from cystectomy sufficiently to allow chemotherapy to start within two months of the operation they will not be eligible.

In this study the regimen has been changed from that of the Phase II study to increase the dose of 5FU. Adriamycin 40 mg/m^2 is given I.V. on Day 1 plus 5 FU 500 mg/m^2 I.V. on Days 2, 3, 4, 8, 15 and 22 of each 28 day cycle, for one year.

Since the study was implemented in 1979 recruitment has been disappointingly slow, in part due to a necessity originally for such P3 patients to have no more than three involved nodes. The entry criteria have now been changed to include any patient without metastases and whose nodes are restricted to the area below the internal iliac bifurcation (category N0-2).

During the same period of time members of the EORTC in the United Kingdom, who have wished to treat bladder cancer primarily by radiotherapy, have undertaken a similar study comparing Adriamycin and 5FU versus no additional treatment following radical radiotherapy for patients with category T3 Nx Mo bladder cancer (Study Coordinator Mr. B. Richards, York, England). This study has now recruited 120 patients of which 101 are evaluable. Its first analysis is expected in October 1980.

CONCLUSION

The Urological Group of the EORTC is optimistic that intravesical chemotherapy offers a good chance of improving the prognosis
in patients with category Ta/T1 bladder cancer. Entry rate to the
previous and current studies reflects this optimism. However the
outlook for patients with invasive bladder cancer is less promising.
Systemic chemotherapy is more onerous than intravesical treatment
and the recruitment to the Phase II studies demonstrates continuing
urological doubt as to the likely effectiveness of the agents so
far evaluated. Despite these problems the prognosis for the patient
with invasive cancer is so serious that it is essential to continue
the evaluation of agents by Phase II studies as rapidly as possible
so that effective adjuvant therapy may be developed.

REFERENCES

1. D.P. Byar, C. Blackard, and VACURG, Comparison of Placebo,
    Pyridoxine & Topical Thiotepa in Preventing Recurrence of
    Stage I Bladder Cancer, Urology 10: 556 (1977).
2. R.J. Cross, R.W. Glashan, C.S. Humphrey, M.R.G. Robinson,
    P.H. Smith, and R.E. Williams, Treatment of Advanced Bladder
    Cancer with Adriamycin and 5 Fluorouracil, Brit. J. Urol. 48:
    609 (1976).
3. F. Edsmyr, T. Berlin, J. Boman, P.L. Esposti, H. Gustafson,
    H. Wikström, M. Duchek, and S. Eksborg, Intravesical Therapy
    with Adriamycin in Patients with Superficial Bladder Tumors,
    in: "Proceedings of the First Conference on Treatment of
    Urinary Tract Tumors withAdriamycin," pp 50 - 57 (1979).
4. H.R. England, J.P. Blandy, and A.M.I. Paris, The Treatment of
    Single and Multiple Papillary Tumours of the Bladder (Ta/T1
    NX MO), in: "Bladder Tumors and Other Topics in Urological
    Oncology," M. Pavone-Macaluso, P.H. Smith and F. Edsmyr, eds.,
    Plenum Press, London and New York, pp 343 - 346 (1980).
5. EORTC Urological Group B, The Treatment of Advanced Carcinoma
    of the Bladder with a Combination of Adriamycin and 5 Fluor-
    ouracil, Eur. Urol. 3: 276 (1977).
6. P.A. Gammelgaard, P. Mogensen, and F. Lundbeck, Bladder
    Instillation of Adriamycin in Multiple Recurrent Non-Invasive
    Papillomatous Bladder Tumours, in: "Bladder Tumors and Other
    Topics in Urological Oncology," M. Pavone-Macaluso, P.H. Smith
    and F. Edsmyr, eds., Plenum Press, London and New York,
    pp 329 - 331 (1980).
7. Y.N. Lee, K.K. Chan, P.A. Harris, and J.L. Cohen, Distribution
    of Adriamycin in Cancer Patients. Tissue Uptakes, Plasma
    Concentration after IV and Hepatic IA Administration, Cancer
    45: 2231 (1980).

8. D. Melloni and M. Pavone-Macaluso, Intravesical Treatment of
    Superficial Urinary Bladder Tumours with Adriamycin, in:
    "Bladder Tumors and Other Topics in Urological Oncology,"
    M. Pavone-Macaluso, P.H. Smith and F. Edsmyr, eds., Plenum
    Press, London and New York, pp 317 - 320 (1980).
9. W.M. Murphy and M.S. Soloway, The Effect of Thio-TEPA on
    Developing and Established Mammalian Bladder Tumours, Cancer
    45: 870 (1980).
10. H. Ono, H. Nakano, N. Hiromoto, H. Nihira, T. Shiraishi,
    M. Hirayama, A. Matsuki, M. Fukushinge, H. Nakatsu, and
    K. Kazio, Fundamental and Clinical Studies of Adriamycin
    on Urinary Tract Cancer, in: "Proceedings of the First
    Conference on Treatment of Urinary Tract Tumors with Adriamycin,"
    pp 77 - 87 (1979).
11. P.R. Riddle, The Management of Superficial Bladder Tumours with
    Intravesical Epodyl, Brit. J. Urol. 45: 84 (1973).
12. P.R. Riddle, Survival in Patients Treated with Epodyl (1968 -
    1978), in: "Bladder Tumors and Other Topics in Urological
    Oncology," M. Pavone-Macaluso, P.H. Smith and F. Edsmyr, eds.,
    Plenum Press, London and New York, pp 333 - 334 (1980).
13. M.R.G. Robinson, M.B. Shetty, B. Richards, J. Bastable,
    R.W. Glashan, and P.H. Smith, Intravesical Epodyl in the
    Management of Bladder Tumors: Combined Experience of the
    Yorkshire Urological Cancer Research Group, J. Urol. 118: 972
    (1977).
14. R.O.K. Schade and J. Swinney, Pre-Cancerous Changes in Bladder
    Epithelium, The Lancet 2: 943 (1968).
15. P.H. Smith, Chemotherapy of Bladder Cancer : A Review, Cancer
    Chemother. Reps. (in press)
16. D.M. Wallace and H.J.G. Bloom, The Management of Deeply
    Infiltrating (T3) Bladder Carcinoma : Controlled Trial of
    Radical Radiotherapy Versus Pre-operative Radiotherapy and
    Radical Cystectomy (First Report), Brit. J. Urol. 48: 587 (1976).

THE PHILOSOPHY OF NATIONAL BLADDER CANCER PROJECT STUDIES

G R PROUT Jr.

Chairman, National Bladder Cancer Collaborative Group A
Massachusetts General Hospital and
Harvard Medical School

The National Bladder Cancer Project is supported by the
National Cancer Institute. Collaborative Group A is the therapeutic section of the Project. The Chairman, Deputy and the
Associate Project Director for Clinical Studies are shown in Table
1, along with the institutions now accessioning patients. Each
institution has a named Pathologist, Radiation Oncologist and a
Medical Oncologist in addition to a Urologist who is the Principal
Investigator. The organization is designed to maximize input and
responsibility to each member. A constitution, publication policy,
a Patient Advocate Committee, a policy for extensive internal group
review of protocols and stringent requirements for quality assurance of data submitted and results reported make up the substance of
the Group. Each discipline has its sub-committee. From these sub-
committees come new hypotheses and the validation of old ones
(Figure 1). This is an hypothesis-generating, longitudinal program
we have conducted for the past six years.

The Group's experience with regard to accession and evaluation
of patients is in press (1) and the contents of the manuscript may
not be divulged because of Group policy. However, as an example,
the patients at the Massachusetts General Hospital may be analyzed
to support certain hypotheses (2). We accessioned 353 patients
between November 1973 and December 1977 (Table 2). Only a fraction of these patients, 56 in all, might be studied to learn how
superficial disease responds to the conventional therapy of transurethral resection (TUR) and fulguration. These were all patients
with their first tumor experience. Obviously, they comprised a
group that might be expected to perform better regarding recurrence,
progression and invasion, since they were <u>new</u> patients. Had they
given evidence of some sinister characteristic inherent in their

TABLE 1

National Bladder Cancer Project and National Bladder Cancer Collaborative Group A

NATIONAL BLADDER CANCER PROJECT

    Project Director: Gilbert H. Friedell, M.D., Chairman, Department of Pathology,
                                      St. Vincents Hospital, Worcester, Massachusetts

    Deputy Project Director: Robert Greenfield, M.D., NBCP, Worcester, Massachusetts
    Associate Project Director: Arthur Hilgar, NBCP, Worcester, Massachusetts

NATIONAL BLADDER CANCER COLLABORATIVE GROUP A

        Chairman: George R. Prout, Jr., M.D., Chief of the Urological
                                    Service, Massachusetts General Hospital, Boston

    Administrative Deputy: Janice Kopp, MBA, NBCCGA, Boston

Accessioning Institutions as at mid-1980:

Johns Hopkins Medical Center, Baltimore, Md.   University of California, San Diego, Calif.
Massachusetts General Hospital, Boston, Mass.   University of Iowa, Iowa City, Iowa
Medical College of Virginia, Richmond, Va.   University of Oregon, Portland, Oregon
Roswell Park Memorial Institute, Buffalo, N.Y.   University of Tennessee, Memphis, Tenn.
Rush-Presbyterian-St Luke's Med Center, Chicago, III   University of Wisconsin, Madison, Wis.
                              Virginia Mason Clinic, Seattle, Wash.

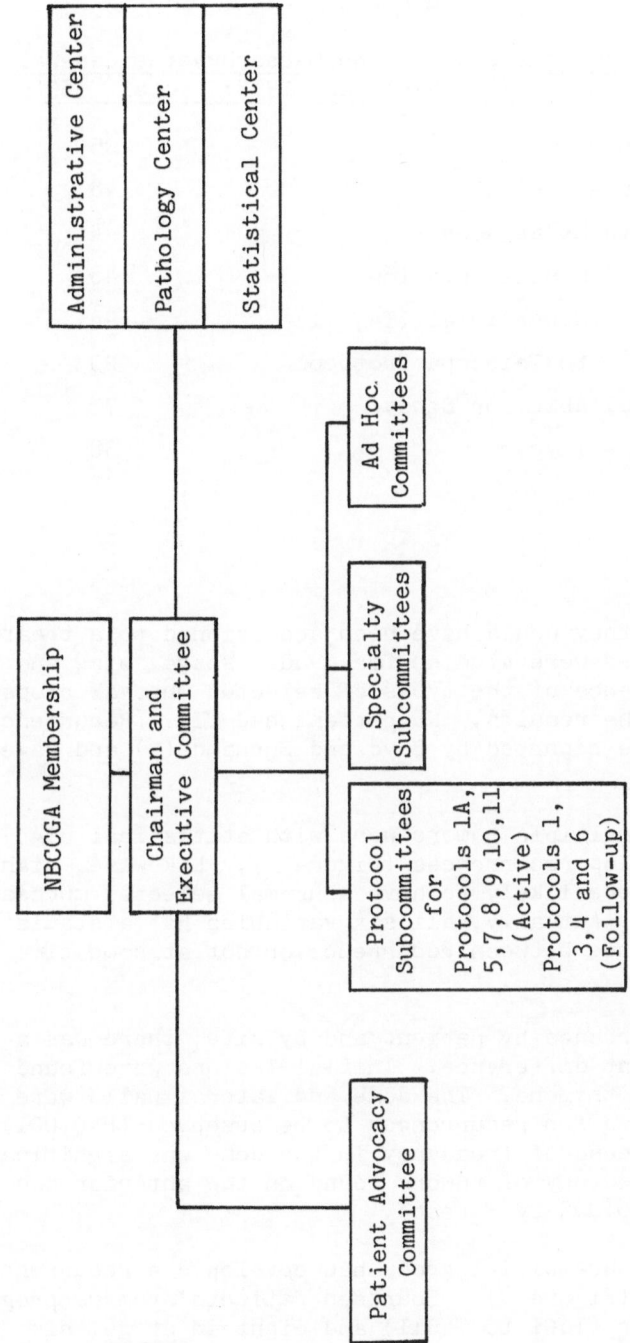

Fig. 1. National Bladder Cancer Collaborative Group A: Organization

TABLE 2

Bladder Cancer Patients seen at the Massachusetts General
  Hospital November, 1973 - December, 1977:   Total   353

Old Patients	205
New Patients	148
Number with Metastases	4
Muscle Invasion	48
Superficial (Ta, T1)	96
to Thiotepa Protocol	25
Number available for Study	71
Follow-up - 1 year	58

disease, i.e. TIS, they would have been accessioned to a treatment
protocol. The tumors were studied for grade, stage, size and multiplicity. The influence of the types of selected mucosal biopsies
was factored into the results. No patient had TIS. Recurrences
were much like those reported by Boyd and Burnand (3) and Page et
al (4).

Patients with multiple tumors were with statistical significance
more likely to develop recurrences (Figure 2). Likewise, higher
grade tumors were more likely to have abnormal selected mucosal
biopsies (Table 3). Actually, all six variables had a statistically
significant difference between recurrence or not at some time in the
patients' courses.

Regarding recurrence by patient and by site, there was a statistically significant difference. Initial lesions were found in
relationship to the trigone. The dome and lateral walls were
greatly favored sites for recurrences to be observed (P<0.001)
(Figure 3). The excess of frequency in the dome was significantly
higher than the frequency of tumors found on the anterior and
posterior walls (P<0.005 by F test).

Nearly 70% of the initial group had developed a recurrence
by the fourth year (Figure 4). Fourteen patients' tumors prog-
ressed; six in grade (TaGI to TaGII) and eight in stage, six
developing muscle invasion (44% of the initial T1 patients).

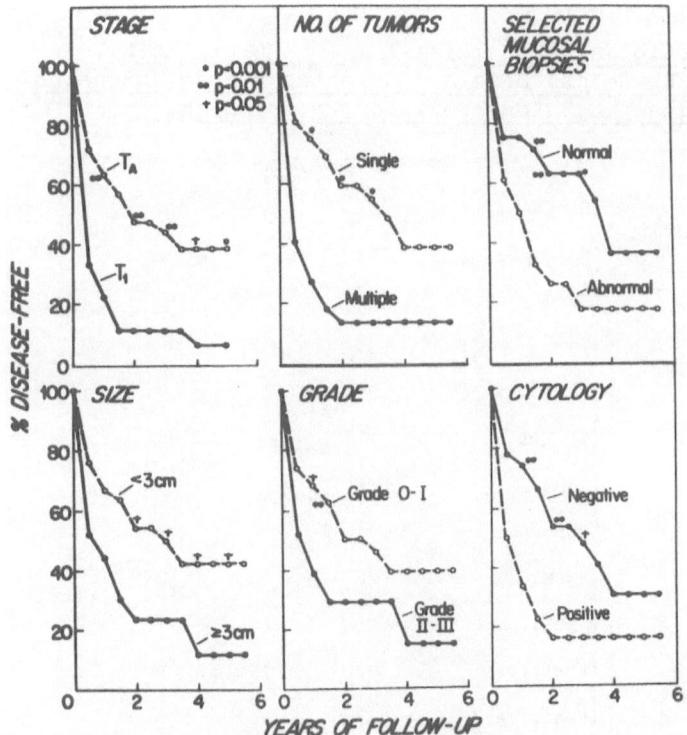

Fig. 2.   Status of Patients in 0 - 6 Years of Follow-Up.

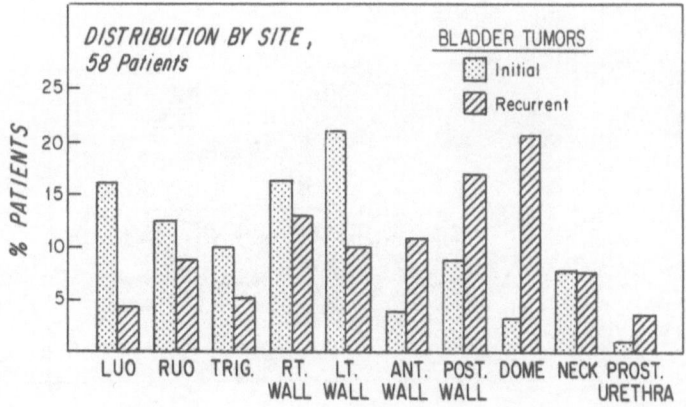

Fig. 3.   Recurrence Sites.

TABLE 3

Prognostic Value of Initial Tumor Multiplicity,
Stage, Grade and Size and Selected Mucosal Biopsies
and Urinary Cytology on Tumor Progression.

		No Progression	Progression	
Multiplicity	(Single	31	5	p < 0.05
	(Multiple	13	9	
Stage	(Ta	39	10	
	(T1	5	4	
Grade	(0-I	27	8	
	(II-III	17	6	
SMB's	(Normal	25	4	
	(Abnormal	11	7	
Size	(3CM	26	7	
	(3CM	18	7	
Cytology	(Positive	12	6	
	(Negative	23	4	

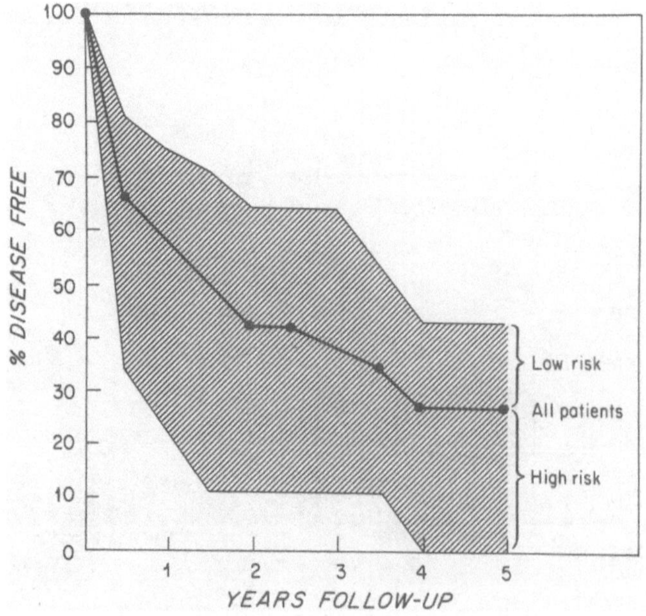

Fig. 4.   Disease-Free Status of Patients, 0 - 5 Years of Follow-up.

Protocol 3: "A Protocol to Determine the Effect of Intravesical Instillation of Antineoplastic Agents on Non-Invasive Primary Carcinomas and the Recurrence Rate of these Carcinomas in Adult Patients".

This study was designed to determine the ablative effect of two doses, 30 or 60 mg, of TTPA on superficial bladder carcinoma, to determine the toxicity of the two doses and to determine if either dose, used prophylactically, would be effective in producing a prolonged tumor-free period (5,6,7). The response rate was 47%, neither dose level produced excessive toxicity, the total being 16%. There were no deaths and four patients were removed because of myelosuppression (Table 4). Dehydration may be important to achieve a response. All patients were treated in the morning after a complete blood count and a platelet count. Treatment continued for four weeks, cystoscopy four weeks later, four more weeks of therapy and a final cystoscopy after four weeks of rest (Table 5). Prophylaxis compared the two doses given fasting on a monthly basis, cystoscopy being carried out every three months for 24 months. The recurrence rate was compared to a control group (Figure 5). It is important to note that this group consisted of a variety of patients, some of whom had been successfully treated with thio-tepa (Table 6). This group, 32% of the total, is referred to as the "post-therapy prophylaxis" group.

When recurrences of the control group were compared with those receiving drug, some advantage for the TTPA group was suggested (Figure 5). When the "post-therapy Prophylaxis" group were removed, the advantage almost disappeared (Figure 6). When this group of patients is compared to the others, it is evident that the great advantage lies with those who have been previously successfully treated (Figure 7). Thus, because the advantage is so great (no recurrence in one year), it seems quite appropriate to leave behind a small Ta lesion to act as an index lesion. If eight weeks of TTPA does not destroy the lesion, then further TTPA for prophylaxis would seem fruitless. On the other hand, if theraputic TTPA destroys the lesion, prophylactic TTPA would seem clearly indicated.

Protocol 4: "Definitive Radiation Therapy versus Adjuvant Radiation Therapy and Cystectomy for Invasive Bladder Cancer", is a Phase III study in follow-up. Between August, 1974, and December, 1976, 100 patients were accessioned; 80 completed the assigned treatment. Analysis awaits long term follow-up.

Protocol 4A was a feasibility study to determine if 4000 rads might be administered to patients with invasive bladder cancer and in whom prompt radical cystectomy might be performed. Fifty-eight patients were so treated. One patient died and the serious complication rate was 6/49 (12%). This study formed the initial steps for Protocol 7 (vide infra).

TABLE 4

Thio-tepa Treatment: Frequency of Observed Toxicity, by Dose

| | OBSERVED PROTOCOL TOXICITY | | | | SUBTOTAL | | TOTAL |
	LEUKOPENIA NO. (%)	THROMBO-CYTOPENIA[†] NO. (%)	URINARY TRACT SYMPTOMS* NO. (%)	COMBINATION[+] NO. (%)	OBSERVED TOXICITY NO. (%)	NO REPORTED TOXICITY NO. (%)	NO. (%)
30 mg. Thio-tepa	1 (2.0)	3 (6.0)	1 (2.0)	3 (6.0)	8 (16.0)	42 (84.0)	50 (100.0)
60 mg. Thio-tepa	6 (13.4)	0 (0.0)	1 (2.2)	1 (2.2)	8 (18.8)	37 (82.2)	45 (100.0)
TOTAL	7 (7.4)	3 (3.2)	2 (2.1)	4 (4.2)	16 (16.9)	79 (83.1)	95 (100.0)

[†] Reported Toxicity
    Leukopenia: WBC < 3000/mm^3
    Thrombocytopenia: Platelets < 100,000/mm^3

* Includes 1 patient with pyuria, hematuria, urinary tract infection; and
  1 patient with hematuria

[+] Includes 1 patient with a low hemoglobin and a urinary tract infection;
  1 patient with lower back pain, mild hematuria;
  1 patient with leukopenia and a low hemoglobin; and
  1 patient with hematuria, CVA.

NOTE: Of the 16 patients with reported protocol toxicity, treatment was terminated for 4 patients and
      interrupted for the other 12.

TABLE 5

Thio-tepa Treatment: Response to First[+]
and Second Courses* of Therapy, According to Dose

TUMOR RESPONSE

Dose and Course	SUCCESS NO.	(%)	FAILURE NO.	(%)	UNKNOWN** NO.	(%)	TOTAL NO.	(%)
30 mg. Thio-tepa								
First Course	35	(70.0)	13	(26.0)	2	(4.0)	50	(100.0)
Second Course	24	(68.5)	5	(14.3)	6	(17.2)	35	(100.0)
Combined	24	(48.0)	18	(36.0)	8	(16.0)	50	(100.0)
60 mg. Thio-tepa								
First Course	26	(57.8)	15	(33.3)	4	(8.9)	45	(100.0)
Second Course	21	(80.8)	4	(15.4)	1	(3.8)	26	(100.0)
Combined	21	(46.7)	19	(42.2)	5	(11.1)	45	(100.0)
ALL PATIENTS								
First Course	61	(64.2)	28	(29.5)	6	(4.3)	95	(100.0)
Second Course	45	(73.8)	9	(14.8)	7	(11.4)	61	(100.0)
Combined	45	(47.4)	37	(38.9)	13	(13.7)	95	(100.0)

[+]Response to First Course: Success = Slight or moderate reduction of
tumor, or complete remission.

Failure = Appearance of new tumor(s);
tumor larger or unchanged.

*Response to Second Course: Success = Complete remission.

Failure = Histological evidence of
remaining or new tumor.

** Includes 4 patients who refused First Course of Therapy; 8
patients who refused or did not receive the full Second Course.
Exclusion of these 12 patients from the analysis increases the
overall success rate to 54%, 57% for the 30 mg. dose and 51% for
the 60 mg. dose.

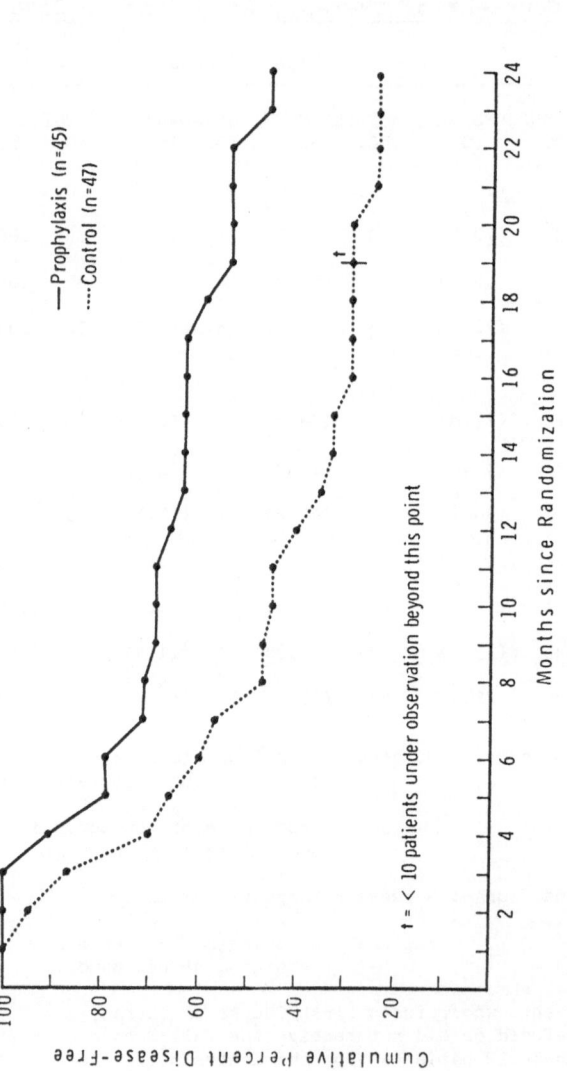

Fig. 5. Thio-Tepa Prophylaxis: Duration of Disease-Free Status – All Patients Entered on Study.

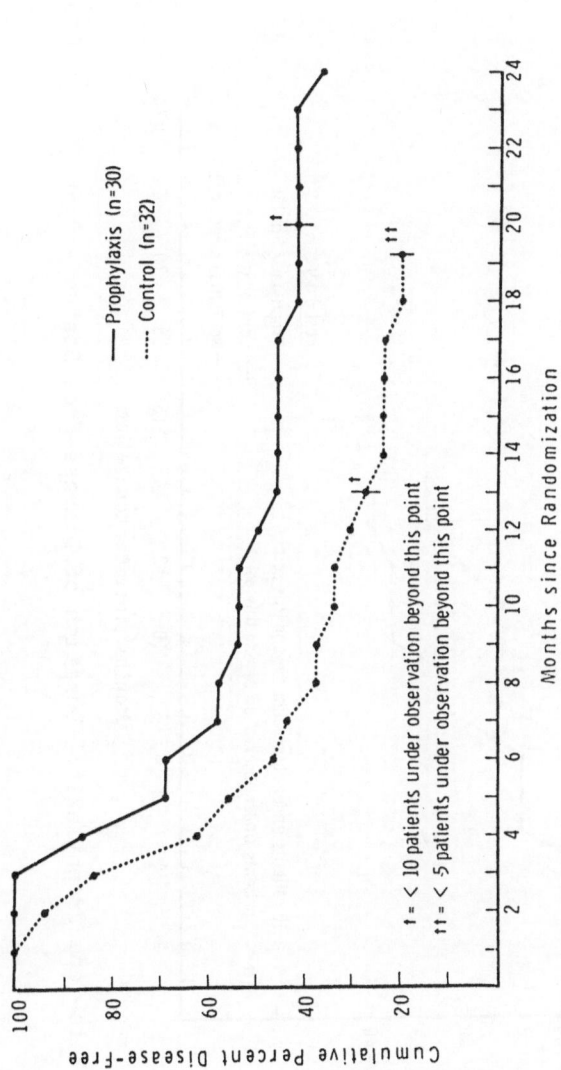

Fig. 6. Thio-Tepa Prophylaxis: Duration of Disease-Free Status - Regular Prophylaxis Group.

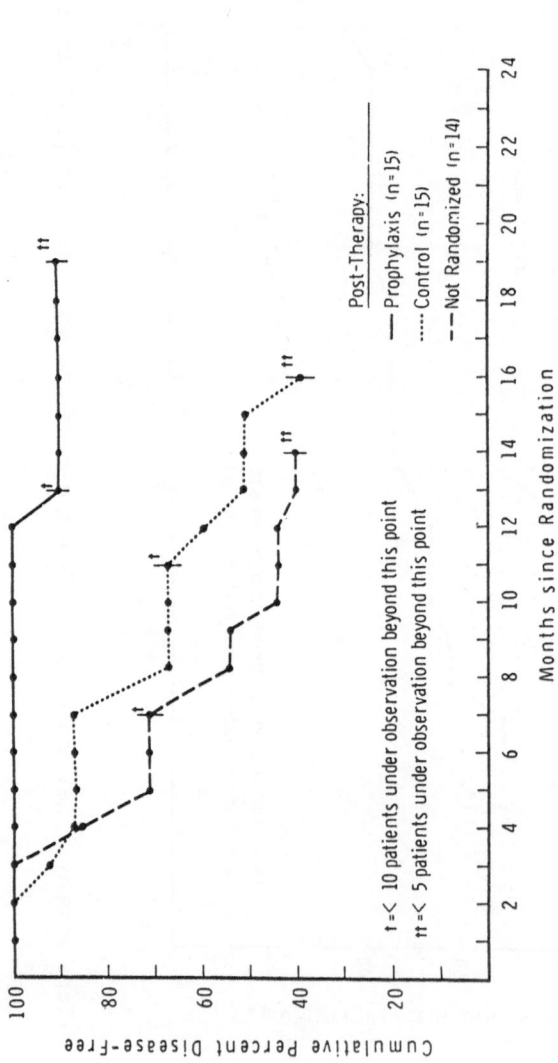

Fig. 7. Thio-Tepa Prophylaxis: Duration of Disease-Free Status – Post Therapy Group.

TABLE 6

Thio-tepa Prophylaxis: Distribution of Patients
by Type of Eligibility According to Assignment

	ASSIGNMENT			
	PROPHYLAXIS			
	30 mg.	60 mg.	CONTROL	TOTAL
PROPHYLAXIS TYPE	NO. (%)	NO. (%)	NO. (%)	NO. (%)
REGULAR				
Three tumor events in past 18 months	5 (21.7)	3 (13.0)	5 (10.6)	13 (14.0)
Multi-focal tumors	5 (21.7)	4 (17.4)	10 (21.3)	19 (20.4)
Investigator's Option	5 (21.7)	9 (39.2)	17 (36.2)	31 (33.3)
SUBTOTAL	15 (65.2)	16 (69.6)	32 (68.1)	63 (67.7)
POST-THERAPY	8 (34.8)	7 (30.4)	15 (31.9)	30 (32.3)
TOTAL	23 (100.0)	23 (100.0)	47 (100.0)	93 (100.0)

Protocol 5 is a Phase III study comparing cis-diamminedichloroplatinum II (CDDP) to CDDP plus cyclophosphamide in patients with advanced, measurable or evaluable bladder cancer (Fig. 8).

All patients will be followed to death to determine response rates, toxicity, disease recurrence and survival rates. Patients with advanced cancer who are, for some reason, ineligible are registered and the reason for ineligibility noted. Thus, a denominator may be obtained. This value provides for some judgement regarding the practicality of such a study, (Fig. 9A,B). This protocol is active and began March 1978.

Protocol 6 is "A Phase I/II Study of Chemical (13-cis-Retinoic Acid) Prevention of Rapidly Recurring Superficial Papillary Carcinomas in Patients Rendered Free of Tumor by Surgical Procedures".

All patients who had a recurrence of low-stage bladder carcinoma within a six-month period and who were rendered free of tumor (demonstrated by histologic biopsy and by cytology) were treated with the orally-administered chemopreventive agent 13-cis-retinoic acid. Treatment was carried out for six months and the patients were to be followed for an additional two-year period. The study

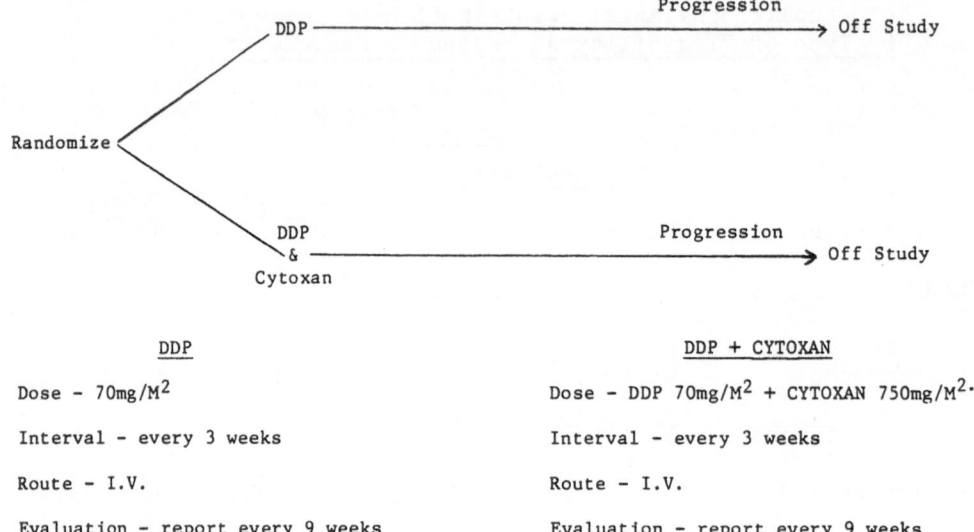

DDP

Dose – 70mg/M^2

Interval – every 3 weeks

Route – I.V.

Evaluation – report every 9 weeks

DDP + CYTOXAN

Dose – DDP 70mg/M^2 + CYTOXAN 750mg/M^2.

Interval – every 3 weeks

Route – I.V.

Evaluation – report every 9 weeks

Fig. 8. Schematic Diagram of NBCCGA Protocol 5

was designed to detect a reduction in the six-month recurrence rate
as compared with historical controls, previously accessioned,
evaluated and followed according to the stipulations set forth in
Protocols 1 and 2.

This study was activated in July, 1978, and was concluded in
June, 1979. Twenty-two patients were accessioned; tumor was found
in four patients at three months and in six at six months. Three
patients were tumor-free at six months. Six patients were withdrawn
due to toxicity, another when the decision to stop accession was
made, and two patients remain unevaluated at this time. Toxicity
included severe pruritis, cheilosis, conjunctivitis, blurring of
vision, elevation of the ESR, progression of Dupuytren's contracture; four of these patients had proven recurrent tumors and
another developed metastases.

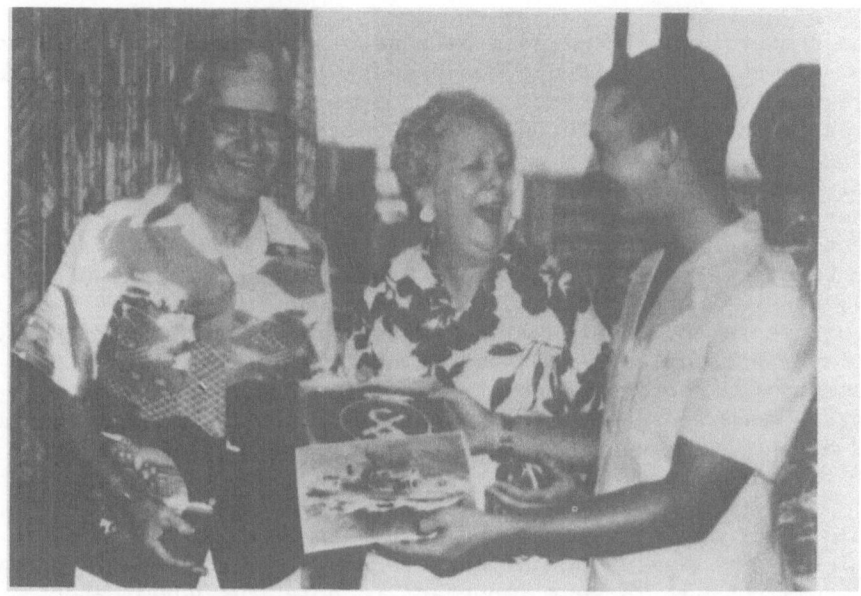

Fig. 9. (A) Photograph of patient (gentleman on left) with neck
         mass of tumor metastatic from bladder (right side of
         photo) (With permission of patient)

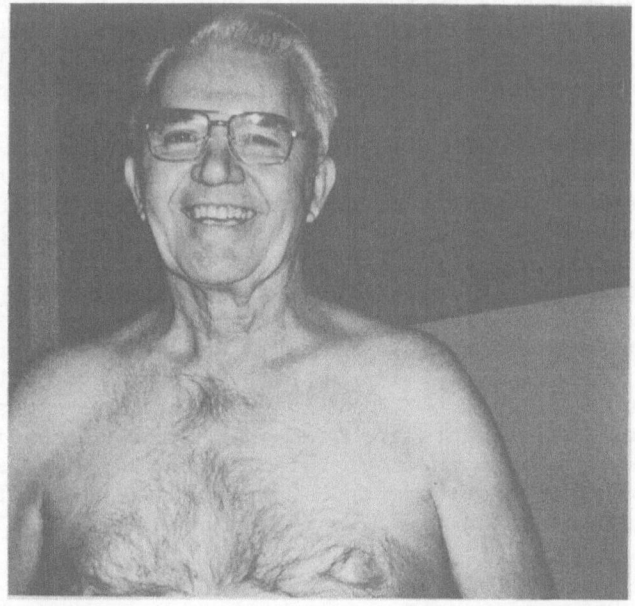

Fig. 9. (B) Photograph of the same patient following CDDP therapy.
         No neck masses were palpable. (With permission of patient)

The protocol was terminated because of the high toxicity rate. However, cis-retinoic acid did not prevent recurrent tumors. This may have been caused by studying a group of patients who were at high risk for developing further recurrences.

Protocol 7 is entitled "Phase III Controlled Study of Adjuvant Chemotherapy (cis-Diamminedichloroplatinum II) Following Preoperative Radiation and Cystectomy in Patients with Invasive Bladder Carcinoma". All patients with histologic evidence of primary, muscle-invasive bladder carcinoma who fulfil the eligibility requirements are treated with preoperative radiation and radical cystectomy. All patients so treated who fulfil the eligibility requirements for receiving chemotherapy are randomized between the adjuvant program for chemotherapy and no further treatment. Eight courses of chemotherapy are administered to the "treatment" group for a five year period.

This study began in November, 1978. As of June 30, 1980, 213 patients were evaluated. Eighty-three were entered and 38 have been randomized. It is very important to note the denominator. Far more patients seem eligible than actually are.

Protocol 8 is a Phase I trial of cis-Diamminedichloroplatinum II (CDDP) combined with small field pelvic radiation therapy for patients with clinical invasive primary carcinoma of the bladder who are unsuitable for cystectomy. This protocol is designed to assess the toxicity associated with concurrent administration of CDDP with small field pelvic radiation therapy by external beam. This study is active, developed this year, and patient accession began in June, 1980.

Protocol 9, "Phase II Master Protocol Evaluation for New Agents for the Treatment of Patients with Advanced Urothelial Cancer", outlines the procedures designed to screen new chemotherapeutic agents for activity in patients having advanced urothelial carcinoma resistant to, or progressing on, treatment with standard agents. A fixed sample size study design will be used, with a stopping rule to avoid continued use of a drug that appears unlikely to meet minimal anti-tumor activity criteria. Sections relating to specific agents will be sequentially incorporated into this protocol as these agents are studied. Phase II studies often make things seem better than they are. The denominators should always be included in such reports. Protocol 9 is ready for the accession of patients, and the first drug to be tested will be M-AMSA.

Protocol 10, a Phase II randomized study to compare the ablative effects of thio-tepa with Mitomycin-C in patients with superficial bladder carcinoma, is undergoing group review. Implementation is expected in the Spring of 1981.

Protocol 11, "Comparative Evaluation of a Single Dose of Intra-
vesical Thio-tepa to an Initial Dose Followed by an Intensive
Maintenance Regimen of TTPA in the Treatment of Patients with
Superficial Bladder Tumor at High Risk of Developing a Subsequent
Tumor", is under group review and activation is expected early in
1981.

REFERENCES

1. S.J. Cutler, N.M. Heney and G.H. Friedell for the National
Bladder Cancer Collaborative Group A: Longitudinal study of patients
with bladder cancer: factors associated with disease recurrence and
progression. In press: J. Urol. 1981.
2. N.M. Heney, B.N. Nocks, J.J. Daly, G.R. Prout Jr.,
J.B. Newall, P.P. Griffin, T.L. Perrone and W.M. Szyfelbein: Ta
and T1 bladder cancer: location, recurrence and progression.
In press: Brit. J. Urol. 1981
3. P.J.R. Boyd and K.G. Burnand, Site of bladder tumor recurrence.
Lancet 3: 1290-1293 (1974)
4. B.H. Page, V.B. Levison and M.P. Curwen, The site of recurrence
of non-infiltrating bladder tumors, Brit. J. Urol. 50: 237-241 (1978)
5. W.W. Koontz Jr., G.R. Prout Jr., W. Smith, W.J. Frable and
J.E. Minnis for National Bladder Cancer Collaborative Group A, The
use of intravesical thio-tepa in the management of non-invasive
carcinoma of the bladder. In press: J. Urol. 1981

CONTRIBUTORS

HELMUTH ADOLPHS
Urologist, Univ. Klinik Urologie, Bonn, DBR.

CHARLES KEITH ANDERSON
Senior Lecturer in Urological Pathology, University of Leeds, UK;
Honorary Consultant Urological Pathologist, Yorkshire Regional
Health Authority.

LENNART ANDERSSON
Professor of Urology Karolinska Institute, Stockholm, Sweden;
Urology expert of the Swedish Ministry of Health; Swedish delegate
of the Société International d'Urologie.

JEAN AUVERT
Professeur à la Faculté de Medecine; Directeur, Service Urologie,
Hôpital Henri Mondor, Creteil, Paris, France.

CHARLES BOUFFIOUX
Specialist Adjoint en Urologie Hôpital Bavière (Prof. C. Macquinay);
Docteur en Sciences Cliniques, University of Liège, Liège, Belgium;
Rédacteur en chef Acta Urologica Belgica.

LOUIS DENIS
Professor of Urology, Vrije Universiteit Brussel, Brussels, Belgium;
Chief, Dept. Urology A.Z. Middelheim, Antwerp, Belgium;
National Coordinator, EORTC GU Group, Belgium.

WALTER DE SY
Professor and Chairman, Department of Urology, University of Ghent,
Ghent, Belgium.

HERMAN de VOOGT
Professor, Vrije Universiteit, Amsterdam, Netherlands; Chief, Dept.
of Urology, Academic Hospital, Vrije Universiteit, Amsterdam.

WILLY GREGOIR
Chief of the University Department of Urology and Prof. of Urology
at the University of Brussels; Honorary Professor of Urology at the
University of Barcelona; General Secretary of the European Association of Urology.

FOLKE EDSMYR
Professor of Oncology and Director Radiotherapy, Karolinska Hospital,
Stockholm, Sweden; Director, World Health Organization Collaborating
Centres for Research and Treatment of Urinary Bladder Cancer.

GUSTAV JACOBI
Oberartz and Faculty Member, Dept. Urology, Johannes Gutenberg
Universität (Prof. R. Hohenfellner), Mainz, Germany.

ALAIN LACHAND
Attaché Hôpital Cochin, Paris, France.

WOLFGANG LUTZEYER
Professor and Chairman Urology, Rheinisch-Westfälische Technische
Hochschule, Aachen, DBR; Co-Editor: Zeitschrift für Urologie,
Der Urologe.

JOSE MARTINEZ-PIÑEIRO
Professor and Chief, Department of Urology, C.S. La Paz, Universidad
Autonoma, Madrid, Spain.

TADAO NIIJIMA
Chief, Department of Urology, University of Tokyo, Tokyo, Japan;
President, Japanese Urological Association.

MICHELE PAVONE-MACALUSO
Professor, Clinical Urology, University of Palermo, Palermo, Italy;
Director, International School of Urology and Nephrology, Erice;
Delegate, International Association of Urology; Chairman, EORTC
Urological Group.

GEORGE PROUT, Jr.
Professor of Surgery, Harvard Medical School, Boston, USA; Chief,
Urological Service, Massachusetts General Hospital; Chairman,
National Bladder Cancer Collaborative Group A, National Bladder
Cancer Project.

HERMAN RUBBEN
Resident in Urology, Department of Urology, Rhein-Westf. Techn.
Hochschule, Aachen, DBR.

CLAUDE SCHULMAN
Chef de Service Urologie, Hôpital Erasme, Université Libre de
Bruxelles, Brussels, Belgium; Editor, European Urology.

PHILIP SMITH
Head of Department of Urology, St. James's University Hospital,
Leeds, UK; Secretary, EORTC Urological Group.

ADOLPHE STEG
Professeur de Clinique Urologique à l'Université René Descartes,
Paris V, France; Chef de Service d'Urologie à l'Hôpital Cochin,
Paris; Rédacteur en Chef des Annales d'Urologie; Membre de l'Executive
Committee of European Urology.

WINFRIED VAHLENSIECK
Lehrstuhl Urologie-Direktor Univ. Klinik Urologie, Bonn, DBR;
Editor, Fortschritte der Urologie und Nephrologie.

BRIGIT van der WERF-MESSING
Professor of Radiation Therapy, Erasmus University, Rotterdam;
Chairman, Dept. of Radiation Therapy, Rotterdam Radio-Therapy
Institute and Erasmus University, Rotterdam, Netherlands;
Chairman, International TNM Committee of the UICC.

RAOUL VEREECKEN
Professor in Urology, Katholieke Universiteit Leuven, Louvain,
Belgium; Co-editor, Urological Research.

ALAN YAGODA
Attending Physician, Solid Tumor Service, Dept. of Medicine, Memorial
Hospital, New York, USA; Associate Professor of Clinical Medicine,
Cornell University Medical College, NYC; Chairman, National Bladder
Cancer Project Confederation; Consultant, Protocol Review Committee,
EORTC Genito-urinary Tract Cancer Cooperative Group.